I0090253

World of Fitness
An Introduction to Body Building

Dashawn Nichol

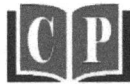

CP

Cadmus Publishing
www.cadmuspublishing.com

Copyright © 2023 Dashawn Nichol

Published by Cadmus Publishing
www.cadmuspublishing.com
Port Angeles, WA

ISBN: 978-1-63751-404-7

All rights reserved. Copyright under Berne Copyright Convention, Universal Copyright Convention, and Pan-American Copyright Convention. No part of this book may be reproduced, stored in a retrieval system, or transmitted in any form, or by any means, electronic, mechanical, photocopying, recording or otherwise, without prior permission of the author.

WARNING: The information in this book is based upon the author's experiences with clients of his own and his experience with himself. No information provided in this book supersedes or overrides any medical advice.

NOTE: This book is intended to target beginners and intermediate-level bodybuilders. It is an introductory book that compares the habits from the humbling fitness lifestyle with its applicability to everyday life. This book will serve as a core introduction to bodybuilding.

Due to this being an introductory book, I will not cover advanced concepts such as posing and dieting for competition nor any competition prep routines and plans. However, I will provide secrets of my own that I used to capitalize on building a better physique. To date, I have a deadlift max of 605lbs, a bench press max of 365lbs, and a squat max of a little over 500lbs. As you will learn shortly, these are the 3 main lifts that help bodybuilders not only measure their strength but prime the composition of the body.

ENJOY!

TABLE OF CONTENTS

PROLOGUE

INSIGHT INTO THE AUTHOR'S DRIVE

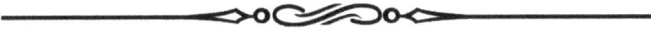

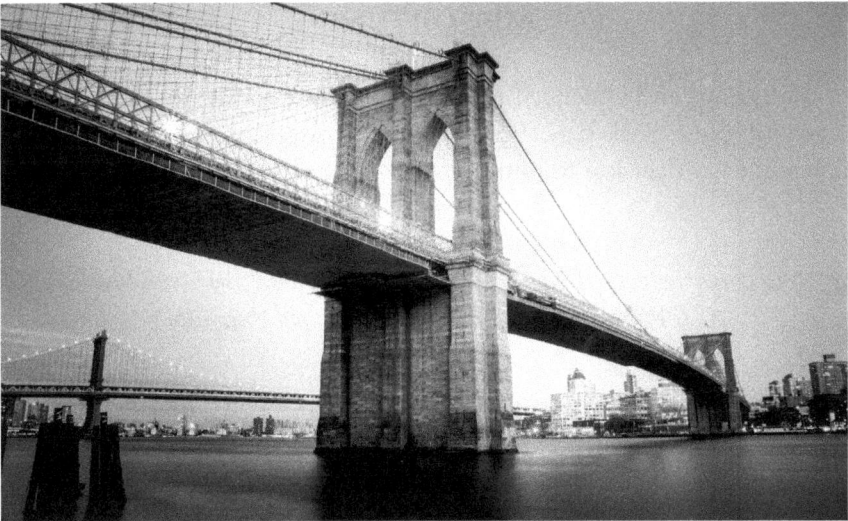

Brooklyn, New York is where it all started. Born and raised. I love my city, but as we all know or have heard, it is a jungle. Survival of the fittest was the way of life, and I wouldn't rather have it any other way.

ACKNOWLEDGEMENT

Growing up as the youngest child in my household, I made it a point to always be recognized for my hard work.

"The deepest principal in human nature is the craving to be appreciated,"
William James.

Along with the chores that were assigned to me, I cleaned the house when my parents were at work and shoveled the snow without being asked. Considering the fact that my parents would eventually ask me to complete those tasks anyway, what made the situation different was my initiative. Being proactive instead of reactive was my nature. This trait was what separated me from my friends, and it allowed me to be less of a burden on my family.

MISFORTUNE

With gangs and violence being second nature to my upbringing in the streets of New York City, I used my early development in behavior to help guide my decision to join the military in pursuit of independence.

"All human situations have their own inconveniences," Benjamin Franklin
(American political leader, scientist, and polymath).

The military was my escape from the risk of ending up dead or in prison. However, after joining the military and completing five years of honorable service, I was convicted at General Courts-Martial (the military's justice system) for crimes I did not commit. Contradictory to the evidence which supports my innocence, on April 10th, 2018, I was sentenced to twenty-five years in prison.

All of my hard work, hopes, and dreams were taken from me the moment the jury announced the verdict. Life as I knew it was practically over. I was now labeled a felon; the very thing I had left NYC to avoid becoming.

Though I suffered from this misfortune, there is something Brooklyn has always taught me. Something that has stuck with me over the years and that is to be prosperous. To NEVER give up. A quarter of a century was my adjudged sentence in exchange for my five years of honorable service and yet, I never gave up. I never gave up on life, my dreams, or my future.

As I continue to fight towards proving my innocence, even with that stigma on my name, giving up will NEVER become an option.

<u>ADVERSITY</u>

I found optimism through fitness. Pessimists see a problem in every opportunity while optimists see an opportunity in every problem.

"Grant me the serenity to accept the things I cannot change, the courage to change the things I can, and the wisdom to know the difference," The Serenity Prayer.

My ambition is what keeps me afloat. Ambition shows that you are willing to work for something. Circumstances change but with great enough ambition, you will overcome those circumstances and work until you reach prosperity. If I gave up, this book would have never made it to your hands. I had to face the reality of my situation.

People get away with committing crimes everyday and innocent people go to prison every day, but such is life. While I resent my current situation, I realize that crying about it more than I already have will only discourage me and bring down my morale. Instead, this is what I use as my source of motivation. To get back and give back.

I will prove to society that I am not the criminal that the military justice system makes me out to be. The military has a famous quote which is "perception is reality," which, in my case, means merely that an allegation is enough to prosecute. Regardless of how things may be perceived, I will continue to fight to get my freedom, future, and life back. I will show people that perception can be a deception.

This book is a direct reflection of the value that fitness has brought into my life while dwelling in the solitude of Fort Leavenworth Prison. Fitness is one of my coping mechanisms and I am willing to help you achieve peace and serenity through the lifestyle that your mind and body deserve. **WHAT IS YOUR EXCUSE?** If you have one, let that be your motivation. Let that drive you. Motivation is of paramount importance. If I can attack my problems head-on without quitting, then you can do the same.

Every journey begins with the first step. Your first step was already taken when you picked up this book. By committing yourself to read this book, you too will learn about the life of fitness from a philosophical perspective. Surely, it will bring to you the same astonishing results it has brought to me.

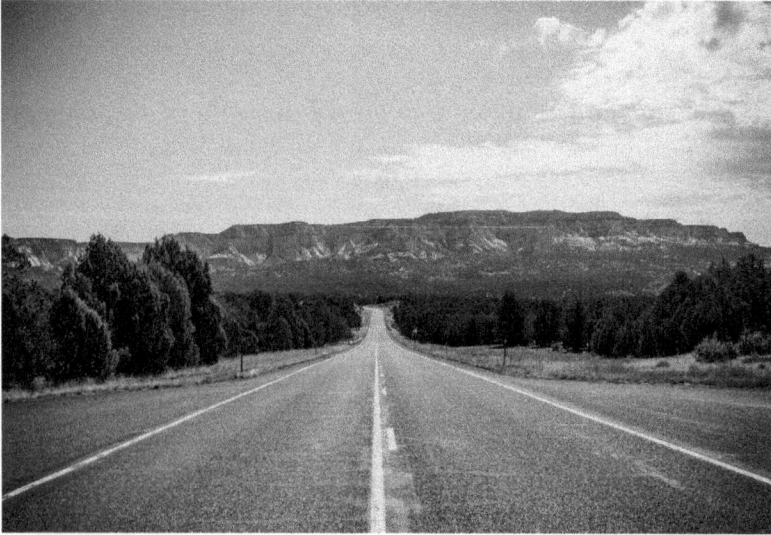

"You have to know where you've been to know where you are going."

INTRODUCTION

———◇○◠◠○◇———

World of fitness will be your primer into the fitness lifestyle. Most textbooks overwhelm the reader with information, making it hard for them to identify key core principals. Understanding a few critically important concepts will provide you with more value than trying to ingest everything about a subject matter.

"If you don't understand something, it is because you don't understand its context," Richard Rabkin (Psychiatrist).

The premise of this book is to provide you with the identity of the most important fundamentals of fitness in a consolidated number of pages. The book's layout is designed to get you acclimated with both the **MENTAL** and **EMOTIONAL** aspects of fitness, before engaging yourself in any **PHYSICAL** activity. For those who are not aware, many people fail to achieve their physical fitness goals because they don't account for the other two most important factors.

First is your mental, which is what helps you to keep going when the weight gets heavy or your body gets tired. Your emotions help when you get flustered because the results you want are not coming as fast as you would like them to come.

World of Fitness is targeted towards those who struggle to commit. It uses real-life examples and real-life scenarios to allow the readers to gain insight into the effects that fitness has in every area of life. Primarily, this book is an introduction to bodybuilding but secondarily, it will provide you with a thought process blueprint that you can use in your everyday life to attack every goal along the way; and it is all done through the life-style of fitness.

WHAT IS FITNESS TO YOU?

To many people, fitness is simply attending the gym and getting, if not staying, in shape. Naturally, people associate the word "fitness" with bodybuilding and aesthetic models that broadcast their muscles. Truly, fitness goes beyond the development of the body. It is a mindset more so than a way of life.

Before	After

A body that stems from this humbling lifestyle is only a fraction of what can be achieved through fitness, but it means a lot. A fit body alone shows that someone has discipline. It shows that someone has dedication, perseverance, and patience and is able to commit to something long enough to reach a goal. This goal becomes one that others would see and want but misjudge how hard it was to achieve.

So, I commend you for wanting change because change is painful. Few people have the courage to change or even seek it until the cost of staying the same outweighs the pain required for change. What people fail to understand, is that realizing a problem before it occurs is the best way to prevent the problem, to begin with.

It shouldn't take lung cancer for a smoker to know enough is enough or diabetes for a person with a medical condition to figure out that they are unhealthy. Unfortunately, it happens. This is simply because people would rather do the same thing over and over again while expecting different results. There is a word for that…it's called "INSANITY." Don't fall victim to it.

"I may not have gone where I intended to go, but I think I have ended up where I intended to be," Douglas Adams (Humorist and Author).

Discipline is one of the key factors fitness can bring into your life. Without discipline, you lack it all. It is essential to recognize the importance of discipline as it is tied into your everyday decision-making skills. This book will magnify your capabilities of building your body to your liking while allowing you to explore and open-mindedly accept the benefits that are attached to the lifestyle's values.

Anything worth working for is worth having. I, myself, have benefitted from the fitness lifestyle in more areas than a bench press or a squat rack. Fitness has helped me overcome financial hardships and contributed greatly towards my *MENTAL, PHYSICAL* and *EMOTIONAL* states of life, but it starts with your mindset. You have to be willing to accept the fact that it will take hard work, commitment, and more importantly, time.

Do not expect immediate results. Relevantly consider how long it took you to get into the position you are in now. One donut did not make you gain all the weight you want to lose, nor did one purchase put you in the amount of debt that you are in, so be patient.

Over the course of this book and with a little patience, you will develop the habits and discipline needed to overcome whatever obstacles life has thrown your way.

<u>INTRODUCTION TO BODYBUILDING</u>

Body building is learned through repetition. Trial and error. With experience, you learn ways to captivate your training and styles for better performance. Training is not just for the looks (though a good incentive). Every part of your life will be positively affected. Self-preservation, confidence, self-esteem, your mental state, your psychological state, your emotional well-being, and even your sex drive. It creates a solid basis for the practice of life's core principles by adding struggle, temptation, commitment, and overdrive, all of which we endure daily.

What it all boils down to is discipline. I titled this book World of Fitness because the commitment to the lifestyle will allow you betterment in what the world has to offer. You will learn the basics of bodybuilding including the composition of the body, primary exercises used by bodybuilders to target individual muscle groups, how to build a workout plan, what training variables are used to assist you in your goal, and much more.

Ask yourself, "is it really worth it?" This is a marathon, not a sprint. Therefore, if you are expecting this to be a cheat code for muscles or a lose weight immediately kind of book, you should put it down because it is not for you.

However, if you are searching for structure in every area of life through fitness, then continue reading and reap the benefits that fitness has to offer by changing your paradigm to a **World of Fitness.**

PART I

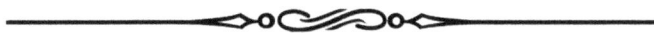

MENTAL

"90% of this game is ½ mental," Yogi Berra (Former Baseball player and Malapropist).

CHAPTER 1

VISION

———————⇌o◠◡◠o⇌———————

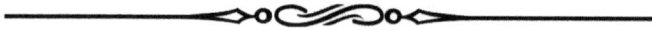

"Before getting acquainted with the physical part of fitness, we will first need to address the mental aspect. This part helps us look at the life subjectively as opposed to objectively. It requires your mind to adopt a state where analytical thinking becomes crucial for every action or decision you make."

Finding your Motivating Factor

Vision is one of the most powerful mental aspects of the fitness lifestyle. In order to have a vision, you must have a motivator. For some people, their motivator is to be able to obtain financial freedom or to overcome a sickness or addiction from which they suffer.

For others, being able to support their family or the pursuit of their dreams may suffice. For me, it's time. Time became of huge importance because so much of it was taken away from me and I won't ever be able to get it back. In retrospect, I use the time that I have productively by doing my best at everything which requires it to be spent.

In turn, your vision is your purpose, and your purpose becomes your motivator. Take some *time* to do some deep, internal searching to find out what it is that motivates you. This may require some critical but mandatory thinking. If necessary, put this book down until you are sure that you know exactly what it is that motivates you.

"Action comes about if and only if we find a discrepancy between what we are experiencing and what we want to experience," Philip J. Runkel (Professor of Psychology).

Lack of Vision

Persistency and consistency are the answers to a lot of problems we as humans face in everyday life. If you learn to use any of your "failures" as lessons, you can benefit from those experiences. Quitting should not be an option. Only people who lack vision quit. I read about an experiment in a book by Joel Osteen about rats and their behaviors. The research developers wanted to test how the rat's attitudes affected their will and desire to live.

They placed one rat in a large container filled with water, making escape impossible. They then placed that container in a room with no light. After timing how long the rat would swim for without giving up, they discovered the rat lasted barely over three minutes. Developers then put another rat in the same container but this time, illuminated a light into the room. This time, however, the rat swam for more than 36 hours.

I am no mathematician, but the difference is "DAY" and "NIGHT." The rat with light swam roughly 700 times longer. This is simply because the rat with no light saw no reason to keep swimming. After all, his vision was intercepted by darkness.

Application of Motivator

When you know what it is that motivates you, it makes it harder to quit. In times of struggle or difficulty, you will remember that there is a reason why you do what it is that you are doing. This would apply significantly when you are working hard to achieve something, but the progress is not coming as fast as you would like for it too. This is why it is important for you to realize that the cause is much bigger than the temporary discomfort you may be experiencing.

No matter what your motivating factor is, you need to use that factor as a drive to succeed in everything that you do. A drive feeds off your motivator by entering your motivator into your vision which in turn builds tolerance and patience. Your drive is what will push you to finish any task you have allotted yourself.

In relation to fitness, the same mindset applies. Without vision, there is no end goal. An example I can give you is push-ups. Imagine doing push-ups and counting upwards, "twenty-one, twenty-two, twenty-three," and so on and so forth. When will the numbers stop? Numbers are infinite. The higher you go, the more the push-ups will hurt. In perspective, this is because there is no finish line in your vision. Now, if I asked you to do fifty push-ups and you counted them down, "eighteen, seventeen, sixteen," magically, you will notice that towards the end, you will have more energy to finish because you know that the end is approaching.

"Great things are not done by impulse, but by a series of small things brought together," Vincent Van Gogh (Artist).

Most battles we face are psychological and able to be overcome. Once you establish your source of motivation, keep it firmly planed in your vision because you will need to identify an achievable goal (discussed in the goal ID chapter) you would like to attain. Often overlooked is the fact that every goal requires small accomplishments along the way.

Small accomplishments are motivators by momentum. Some of us have heard this saying before, but for those who have not, it goes; "How does one eat an elephant? One bite at a time." After completion of each small accomplishment, you will build courage going into your next challenge, ultimately leading to the end goal.

Under-estimation.

A lot of people fall short of their goals because they fail to acknowledge the small accomplishments associated with the goal. This failure of acknowledgment attacks their patients, resulting in a negative impact on their motivation. Identifying the smaller accomplishments in a goal's process prevents underestimation before commitment.

To elaborate a little more, seeking employment would be a prime example of this. There is a definitive process that goes with doing that. You will first have to draft, edit, and revise a resume illustrating your credentials. Next, you will need to fill out a job application for your desired position. Many people may think that the process ends after acceptance, but it does not.

In many cases, you will have to attend a job interview for the intended position and if hired, possibly conduct OJT (on-the-job training) to familiarize yourself with the company and its policies. This is all done prior to receiving your first pay-check. Breaking down a goal into smaller accomplishments allows you to properly identify a process and prepare, leaving little to no room for intimidation during the time of execution. Use the small accomplishments as mile stones on your journey.

Whether your goal is to get fit, pay off debt or get a college degree, just do it. A vision starts with an idea of who you are now and who it is you want to be. Yes, it is going to take some hard work! Any meaningful goal will require dedication, desire, determination, and discipline. I am here to tell you that procrastinating any longer will not make the process any easier. Invest in yourself, your life, and your future because the permanent benefit outweighs the temporary discomfort.

Before continuing to Chapter 2, stand in front of a mirror and take a look at yourself. Look yourself in the eyes and say, "I take you seriously…**I Take You** Seriously...**I TAKE YOU SERIOUSLY!**" Remember, in order to adopt the fitness mindset, you first have to be receptive to the information provided in this book. So, don't cheat yourself, go find that mirror!

After you have accepted the challenge of commitment towards change, write some of your immediate goals down on the chart provided below, and then, sign the commitment box to self. These goals will later be re-identified in chapter six, modified, and properly executed as a plan will be formulated to aid in completion. Once you have signed the commitment box, allow one person, either a friend or a family member to oversee your goals and hold you accountable by recognition with their signature.

GOALS	SMALL ACCOMPLISH-MENTS
Goal 1:	SA1: SA2: SA3:
Goal 2:	SA1: SA2: SA3:
Goal 3:	SA1: SA2: SA3:

WORLD OF FITNESS COMMITMENT

I, _____ (INSERT NAME)
HEREBY PROMISE MYSELF THAT STARTING TODAY
_____ (INSERT DATE). I WILL SET TIME ASIDE
FOR MYSELF TO ACCOMPLISH MY GOALS LISTED ABOVE.

I ACKNOWLEDGE THAT BY SIGNING THIS, I AM OBLIGATING MYSELF TO THE DUTY OF COMPLETING MY SMALL ACCOMPLISHMENTS IN ORDER TO ATTAIN MY GOALS.

NAME ABOVE SIGNATURE

_____

WITNESS SIGNATURE

_____

Lastly, repeat after me:

"WHAT I BREAK, I WILL FIX."

"WHAT I START, I WILL FINISH."

"WHAT I SEEK, I WILL FIND."

"WHAT I WISH TO BE, I WILL BECOME!"

CHAPTER 2

STANDARDS

———◇○〰◇○◇———

It is absolutely mandatory that you implement standards into your everyday life. A *standard* is a tool of measurement to assure that you are applying the necessary effort to attain a goal or maintain a status. Higher standards usually result in higher accomplishments. It is scientifically proven that if you raise a standard, people will try to apply the necessary amount of will power to meet that standard. This is because people naturally fear failure.

"High achievement always takes place in the framework of high expectation,"
Charles Kettering (Prolific inventor and former head of research for general
motors).

Again, a standard is set in accordance with a goal. Generally, people who set a standard are rewarded. Let us use a race, as an example. The goal of a race is to finish before your competitors. In a race with ten people, only the top three will receive a reward. The standard was set by the 1st person, followed by the 2nd, then the 3rd. Notice that if you take the last two letters out of fir(st), seco(nd), and thi(rd), you will get STNDRD. Pronouncing that would amount to "STANDARD."

You are your own competition, so you set the standard for yourself. Anything that you have to spend time on should merit your best effort. You should always look forward to progressing. If you do twenty push-ups today, do twenty-one tomorrow, and then twenty-two the next day. Holding yourself to prestigious standards contributes towards raising your value (discussed later).

AVOID SHORTCOMINGS

At no point in time should you ever set your standard to the bare minimum. Imagine taking a test that grades from 0-100 with a 65 being a passing grade. What do you think you should aim for? If you thought anything less than 100 then you are wrong. Aim for 100, 100% of the time. It is the metaphor of "aim for the stars so if you fall short, you land on the moon." You do not want to aim for a 65

"HEIGHTEN YOUR STANDARDS"

because if you fall short, you fail. The same mentality applies during exercise.

Your standards are what set you apart from your competition. Let me reiterate that along with others, you are your own and your best competition. Though the standards implemented vary per situation, people will generally hold you to a standard once it is set. Mercedes-Benz advertises itself as a luxurious car brand. They are obligated to uphold the highest standard of quality for their vehicles. Anything short of this will be detrimental to their brand, upsetting their customers.

Quality can entail updated technology, premium material used for the interior, or even durable tires with nitrogen. You will never find a Mercedes that requires regular gas to operate. They all require premium gasoline.

Be aware that if you do not meet or maintain a standard, there are consequences and repercussions. Standards for activities, whether physical or academic wise are set at entry level. These standards are put into place to determine who is actually qualified for participation by attendance. Harvard University for example requires potential candidates to have a GPA of at least 3.9 weighted-4.15 unweighted for acceptance alone. While in attendance, all students must maintain the standard of grading to ensure their enrollment within the college. A standard once set must be upheld.

Now, of course, this is a fitness book and I understand that some people may be wondering "when are we going to get to the physical part of fitness?" Though this book is designed to be a significantly quick read for motivation, it is also life changing. The foundation for understanding the fundamentals of the lifestyle is crucial. We will get to the physical part of fitness but when we get there, we should see life through a different paradigm.

"You can get anything you want in this life if you help enough other people get what they want," Zig Ziglar (Sales Guru).

I have a standard that I hold myself dear to and it includes teaching and helping others understand what it is that they do not. My belief is centered on the fact that if you do not mentally and emotionally prepare for this lifestyle, you will not make it long enough to reap the complete benefits of fitness. So, that standard is set now.

If you do not set standards, you will be misjudged by others. Failure to identify the standards that you want to live up to can cause misrepresentation of yourself. Far too often, people live up to what they believe may be someone else's standard. We see or hear about it all the time. People go into debt to purchase a vehicle they cannot afford or buy clothing and jewelry outside of their budget. They believe that in order to be accepted, nice luxurious items are necessary.

That is a standard that they believe other people will hold them to. Really, what is taking place is a misrepresentation. They are overwhelming themselves with a financial crisis by applying a standard of wealth to impress others. Instead, the standard you set for yourself could have been implemented and upheld so others will not misinterpret or misjudge. Your standard of living should not exceed your living standards!

"The limits of my language are the limits of my world," Ludwig Wittgenstein (Philosopher and logician).

You are your own competition, so you are the standard. Maintain a standard of excellence and perfection by doing everything to the best of your ability.

SOCIAL CIRCLE

Once you set a standard, you will notice that you attract like-minded people. Your surroundings will compliment your standard. Statistically speaking, people who survive on fast food are typically overweight. So, if you are looking for a Victoria's Secret model, don't go to McDonald's.

Raising your standards may change your social circle. However, if your friends do not recognize and support your efforts to improve your lifestyle mentally, emotionally, or physically, then they were not good friends to begin with. A friend will help motivate you toward your goal. If you are trying to save money, do not associate with people who always party and go shopping. If you want to lose weight, do not socialize with people who want to drink booze and eat take out. Instead, attract yourself with those on the same mission as you by holding yourself to your standard. Don't just read the words on these pages.

"People don't realize how a man's whole life can be changed by one book,"
Malcolm X (Human rights activist).

Actually, apply it to your life for the better good. It is going to be hard at first because of the separation created by what change is easy? Each chapter you read will expose your mind to a general way of thinking for success. Allow change to take effect in your life by applying standards to every aspect of it. You can do it and you will do it because you have a standard to uphold and that standard is YOU!

CHAPTER 3

VALUE

Everything that you allow to enter your life comes with value attached to it. The value may be monetary, spiritual, sentimental, or just valued by its worth. Whatever the value may be is what allows you to have a connection with that certain item, person, or service. The fitness lifestyle encourages you to place value in *everything* you have, want, or need. By doing this, you will learn to place value in yourself, the people you surrounded yourself with, and the process of whatever journey it is you choose to endeavor.

The value that fitness has brought into my life personally is unbelievable. To say the least, fitness has helped me to cope and stay sane during my incarceration, allowed me to properly educate myself through exercising the mind (reading) as well as obtained my fitness goal physically. Through fitness, I was able to achieve almost any and every goal that I set. So, not only do I value the mindset that the lifestyle encourages, but I also value the hard work and experience it brings with each journey.

LAZINESS

The problem with society today is that people are lazy. They lack the ambition it takes to work hard to achieve what it is they want. If something becomes of value to them, they will cheat or shortcut their way to obtain whatever it is they desire. For the people who actually work hard to acquire what they want, their hard work is overlooked by the falsity that surrounds them taking even credit.

For example; obviously one of the ways hard work is displayed through fitness is from the structure and development of the body. Due to the up rise in surgeries for body enhancements and the use of steroids to promote body growth, the natural physique and development of the body almost goes unnoticed. Unfortunately, the shortcuts that these men and women are indulging in can lead to health issues as life progress which goes directly against the values that fitness is supposed to provide in your life. On a day-to-day basis, that man or woman with the banging body is receiving the same amount if not more praise and compliments than the person who worked hard for their body.

"I can and I will because I am the standard!" Dashawn Nichol (Author of World of Fitness).

THE DIFFERENCE

There will always be easier alternatives to achieve a goal, but a lot is missed by taking the short road. First off, you need to value your body. You only get one for a lifetime. Secondly, when you work for something, its value provides a specific kind of pride and ego you couldn't get if it was given to you effortlessly.

"Value is not intrinsic. It is not in things. It is within us; it is the way in which man reacts to the conditions of his environment," Ludwig Von Moses (Austrian Economist).

By working for something, you become aware of how hard it was to achieve, making it less likely that you will want to lose it. You have probably heard stories about people who have hit the lottery and then gone broke again. It is not because they are stupid (well, that is half the reason), but it is simply because they did not work for that money. See, the people who work for something learn the do's and don'ts along the journey.

Typically, if something is given to you, you would lack the knowledge and experience on what it took to obtain it. You may go to college and cheat your way through, plagiarize your essays and copy a friend's homework. You may still eventually get a degree, but you will lack the knowledge, experience, and challenges that those tests and essays would have prepared you for. Give your life the value that it deserves.

BIRDS OF A FEATHER…FLOCK TOGETHER

As the previous chapter mentioned, you may need to distance yourself from some of your friends during this lifestyle makeover. The friends you do decide to keep will need to be evaluated. What I mean by that is that you will need to identify what kind of value each friend provides to you in your life. It sounds selfish, but realistically, everyone you have allowed to enter your life provides some form of value to it.

It is your duty to identify what that value is for each person.

"Price is what you pay. Value is what you get," Warren Buffet.

I have friends that I can call to party. That is the value they provide in my life. I will not call them for anything other than partying and to make sure they are still alive. When I associate with them in my life, the memories will always be just that…partying. Same for my friends that play basketball or even the ones that make me laugh. If I'm down and need a good laugh, I know exactly who to call and if I want to play ball, I have a long list I can pick from.

The moral of the story is that you will not be able to implement a friend into every aspect of your life because they may not be capable of providing any value in each area. Your doctor can save your life but that does not mean that you should ask him for legal advice. Identify the value of all of your friends.

VALUE YOUR MOTIVATOR

Value is what we base the majority of our decisions off of. The value of your motivator has to be of high value to you. This is what helps people overcome temptation and make choices that contribute towards their goals. If you can place something in your life that you value more than your motivator, then you need to go back to Chapter 1 and re-evaluate what your motivator is before continuing your reading.

For the sake of an example, I will pick on a smoker once more to elaborate on my point. A smoker will always tell someone who does not smoke not to smoke. It is not because they want all the cigarettes in the world to themselves, but it is because they know what low value it encompasses. Even they themselves feel as if the risk is not worth the reward but they value a cigarette more than their motivator if they even have one. So, of course they cannot quit.

I will be the first to tell you that as long as they value the buzz they get from that cigarette; they will continue smoking until they find a motivator. When you are aware that something is not bringing value to your life, you must immediately let it go. Accepting responsibility is the first part towards growth. Being delusional will leave you vulnerable, mentally. Those people who struggle to overcome temptation need to pick up books like this one to understand that a mass of battles toward resistance is mental.

It is hard to sell books that teach the necessities of hard work, discipline, and value however, books like this create hope of value.

"Selling to people who actually want to hear from you is more effective than interrupting strangers who don't," Seth Godin.

The lottery makes hundreds of millions every day by selling people a false sense of hope. This book is not the lottery. In fact, it is the exact opposite. It is a tried-and-true method to help you overcome any obstacle that life throws at you by applying a fitness mentality. This lifestyle encourages the use of intellect as opposed to false hope and blind faith.

"Strive not to be a success, but rather to be of value," (Albert Einstein).

VALUE YOUR BODY-THE PROCESS-AND YOUR VALUES

Place value in your body. The better you treat your body, the better your body treats you. Your body is what is going to carry you to the physical goal that you are trying to reach. When you value something you use it more diligently. Injuries are always possible but become less likely if you first understand the importance of treating your body well via rest, nutrition, stretching, etc. placing uncompromisable value on it.

Value the process. The process is what prepares you for your end goal. Lastly, value your values. It is up to you to continue to fulfill your dreams and goals. Nobody or nothing can stop you once your vision kicks your motivator into your mind.

I value life a little more now being that a large fraction of my own was taken from me. My dream is to help as many people as possible through fitness and its lifestyle using *World of Fitness* as my testament. Unfortunately, I can sell a million books and there will still be seven billion people that remain uneducated about the lifestyle. Still, I use my valuable time to provide guidance to those who decide to take that journey. Now, it is up to you to value the information provided for your use and pass it on to those you value. Anything you value, you shall invest in.

When you invest in your income, you become wealthy!

When you invest in your education, you become wise!

When you invest in your body, you become healthy!

BUT

When you invest in your life, you become it ALL!

PART II

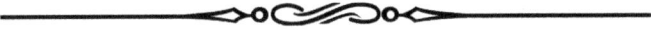

EMOTION

"Control your emotions because it is such which allows our actions to manifest our destiny," Nichol Dashawn (Author of World of Fitness).

CHAPTER 4

CONFINEMENT

———o⌒◯⌒o———

"The emotional part of fitness correlates directly with the mental aspects of fitness. When you have a VISION with STANDARDS that you VALUE you will become attached emotionally to those principles. This section will help you identify and control your emotions which in turn will allow you to identify pitfalls and avoid them."

Re-Defining Confinement

Overlooking the fact that this book was written behind prison walls, confinement goes beyond incarceration. Many people are oblivious to the realization that they are actually confined in more ways than one. So many are confined by a marriage that they have been trying to terminate, a debt or debts they cannot seem to get rid of or even a job that they do not necessarily like but "need" to make income.

According to the Merriam-Webster Dictionary, confinement is defined as "(1) to hold within a location and (2) to keep within limits." Regardless of the different variations of confinement, the fact still remains the same. You are in a situation that *USUALLY* you are trying to unbind from with a grace of hope and a leap of faith. I use the word usually because, again, the type of confinement varies in context. It can be good, or it can be bad. If you have a daily routine, you can confine yourself to the strict terms of that routine. It does not mean that you want to detour from the routine but instead that you hold yourself dear to it.

"We are what we repeatedly do. Excellence then is not an act, but a habit,"
Will Durant (Historian and Philosopher).

People are naturally confined to a mindset that is triggered by their morals and principles developed throughout the course of their lives. What the fitness lifestyle provides is a structure needed to unbind and overcome the negative types of confinement that you suffer from using intellect as opposed to raw knowledge and blind faith.

Raw Knowledge and Blind Faith Misleads

Raw knowledge provides you with a false sense of direction. Each of us grew up differently so each of our morals and principles will differ. What those morals and principals help us to do is create judgment to fill in the gaps to questions to which we do not have the answers.

Generally, when we do not know something, we do research to find guidance. This research may be generated from friends or family, a stranger, a book, or the internet; all of which have the potential to point us in the right direction. However, if the task seems too easy, we allow ourselves to tackle it without identifying the best method of approach.

For example, this is like being locked outside of your house because you lost the key so you break a window for entry, not noticing that the window was not locked, to begin with. Now, you're out of a window and still do not have a key. Here is where we as people apply what I like to call "raw knowledge." We will use our past experiences, context clues or hints, generally inferred instructions, or even straight out copy what we see someone else doing with an "if it works for them it must work for me," mentality.

But this mentality is flawed. I cannot tell you how many times I have witnessed someone walk into the gym with a plan contradictory to the goal they are trying to achieve. These types of people will perform the exercises incorrectly which in turn stagnates their progress and risks injury. Eventually, these people give up because not only do they not know what they are doing, but they do not know why what they are doing is not working. Having inadequate knowledge of a particular subject can leave too much room for interpretation.

"Not knowing how to do something is bad if you're doing it anyways. Not knowing why you're doing something is worse if you're doing it anyways."

Both literally and figuratively, confinement can be identified as a restriction from freedom. It is what prevents one from walking away from that marriage or overcoming an addiction or bind to those credit card payments. In the literal sense, it prevents you from living your life how you desire to live it. Emotional feelings are attached to each kind of confinement based on these wants and desires. Again, do not associate the word with negative feelings. As I said before, when someone says the words, "I DO," they are entering a form of confinement by a marital bond to their spouse. Yet, it is one of the best days of life for some people and it can be seen as a curse to others who may want a divorce.

Remember, the fitness lifestyle encourages, promotes, and demands you look at things subjectively as opposed to objectively. Look for the good in every situation and how to positively effect a negative situation. Using myself as an example, this experience has helped me to grow substantially as a person. Though it constricts and restricts me, it saved me from self-destruction. It deterred me from drinking and smoking. It allowed me to obtain my fitness goal, finish a degree and publish the very book that is sitting in your hand.

I used my time to sharpen my mind through reading and I am served three meals a day. I can name some people who are not incarcerated and who are going through a lot worse. They may not know where their next meal is coming from. I am in no manner promoting incarceration as a positive thing, but life can always be a lot worse. It is the angle at which you look at things. You can look at the glass as half empty or half full. Half full sounds like you are trying to acquire a full cup, while half empty sounds as if something is missing or lost.

Realize that this lifestyle will take a substantial amount of time out of your day. This is something that has to be on your mind subconsciously without actually thinking about it. The decisions you make whether at home, school, or work all effects your progress in this lifestyle. There will be a time when you want to do something, but you know it will be contradictory to the goal that you have set for yourself.

This is when your will power is supposed to guide you in the right direction. This is why I call this chapter confinement. You must confine yourself to the codes of conduct and realize that your goal is more important than any temporary discomfort you may be experiencing. Every time you compromise your goals for temporary satisfaction, you are slowly dissipating the discipline the lifestyle is supposed to instill into you. With a lot of practice, this discipline will become normal behavior.

You will not crave the old habits that you once had because you learned to supplement them with new ones. Better ones at that. Before indulging in the fitness lifestyle, first, you need to understand what it consists of through research and ask yourself if that is what you want. Are you truly going to be able to confine yourself to the codes of conduct required to reap the fruits of the lifestyles labor? Agreeing to confine to the lifestyle is agreeing to base your decisions and actions on rationality, research, and reasoning instead of blind faith and raw knowledge. Unbind yourself from any negative confinement that you may suffer from because **emotions** cloud **mental** contractions which lead to making **physically** impulsive decisions.

Prior to addressing any kind of negative confinement, find out what would be the best method of approach. Clearing up all binds will prevent the negative confinement from hindering your success with a commitment to this lifestyle.

CHAPTER 5

ATTITUDE

A huge part of the fitness lifestyle is learning how to control our feelings, emotions, and **ATTITUDES.** Your attitude will determine if you approach a situation logically or emotionally. Controlling these aspects of your life is mandatory for growth and progression. Changing your attitude will take time. As long as you stay motivated, you will possess the ability to change your attitudes.

ABILITY-is what you are capable of doing

MOTIVATION-determines what you do

ATTITUDE-determines how well you do it.

The attitude you display towards committing to the fitness lifestyle is shown through the results of your transformation. Specifically, it is the attitude that you have for a craft or lifestyle that will determine the amount of hard work, research, time, and energy you will invest into its process. When you become passionate about something, it becomes a part of who you are and what you represent.

That is what authenticates the process needed to achieve the goal you set out to accomplish. The people around you will notice that you are actively engaged in a specific lifestyle because it will be something you display through both your actions and will be something you constantly speak about. Take for instance a religious person. They will always recommend that you pray for necessities and wants or to thank a higher being for the blessings that you receive. They will preach about how good their higher being has been to them and all else that the lifestyle entails.

This is because they are actively engaged in that specific walk of life. Speaking about the journey with others will not only show you have a positive attitude towards a certain type of living, but it will also reiterate to yourself that what you're doing has a purpose behind it. While you constantly teach others about what it is that you believe and are engaged in, you also remind yourself of the commitment that you made to take on the challenge of living said lifestyle, which helps you stay true to the code of conduct.

When it is time for me to eat, exercise, or even complete a task, my behaviors and decisions are consistent with the lifestyle of fitness. I do all my duties with 100% commitment and persistence. This is how it will be when you enter that weight room.

"Always and never are two words that you should ALWAYS remember to NEVER use," Wendell Johnson (Psychologist).

Positive Re-enforcement

If you approach a situation or a goal with a negative attitude, you will not put for your full effort, limiting your potential. "I can't," or "I don't know if I can," are examples of negative attitudes. Believe it or not, this has a major effect on you when you are lifting wights.

"Whether you think you can or can't, you're right," Henry Ford.

Your attitude needs to provide some form of affirmation. Your discouraging attitude will lead you to believe mentally that you lack the capabilities to achieve your goals physically. "I can," and "I will," should be added to your vocabulary. These words will help build assurance. These are words of encouragement. Failures in fitness and life itself should be viewed as steppingstones to access and measure progress. This means that your approach should never entail fear of failure.

What positive re-enforcement provides for you is a sense of security. Positivity is a confidence booster. To put it into perspective, I will use one of my past experiences.

REAL STORY:

I was working out at Planet Fitness one time when a group of three young men entered the gym, all excited and hyped up. If you do not know, Planet Fitness operates under a "non-intimidation zone" policy, so immediately they gained unwanted attention from practically everyone with the amount of noise they were making. The change in the environment seemed to aggravate some people, but I just continued my workout.

During my rest period, I noticed the three men preparing to use the smith machine to do bench presses. At that moment, my current max was 295 lbs. I had been stuck at that number for roughly three months with no idea as to why I could not progress. After a few warmup sets, the first guy attempted my max, completing if for a total of five repetitions. Instantly, my interest was captured. By no means were these guys, "muscle heads" or even bigger than me for that matter, but after the second guy completed the same amount of weight for two repetitions, I was convinced that something had to change.

The last guy being the smallest out of the group also attempted the lift. Impressively, he also completed the lift. At this moment, my workout stopped because I was in awe. Moving along, the first two guys attempted 315lbs, successfully completing it for one repetition. The third guy attempted the lift as well as we all encouraged him. Although he did not complete the lift, the attempt was impressive, being that the weight actually came off his chest before he needed help.

Fortunately, his positive attitude toward the situation made me see what it was that I was missing. He was satisfied even though he failed the lift because come to find out, 295lbs happened to be a new record for him. This reiterated to me that I need to stop being intimidated by the weight and just do it.

Now, I could have been upset like the other gym-goers about these guys coming into the gym, making noise, and having the audacity to make my max weight look too easy but my attitude was the complete opposite.

I took the energy they were giving off and used it to my advantage. I asked the first guy since he was clearly their trainer if he would mind me attempting 315lbs. I told him 295 was my max and he replied "not today," as he encouraged me to attempt the lift. Luckily for me, it was chest day and my muscles were already warmed up. I got under the weight, unracked it, and lowered it to my chest. After the bar contacted my chest, I heard the three men cheering, "push…push…push" as I pressed the bar back up. The rest was history. For the first time ever, I had managed to bench press 315lbs after being stagnated for months.

Always go into a challenge with a winning mentality. Never settle for less. Believe in yourself. That day, I learned that my attitude controlled my destiny. Build a positive attitude prior to engaging in your workout. This can be done through conversation, meditation, music, videos, or even by other people. Positive attitudes are contagious. I could have allowed my fear of failure to overcome my pride and not even attempted the lift to save myself from a potentially embarrassing situation, but I did not. Prior to that day, my attitude had been "I know I can't lift it but let me try it anyway," but looking forward, I know that tackling your goals with confidence will produce the best results.

EXCUSES

Too often do I see people lose before even trying something because their emotions and fear of failure interrupt their desire to win. Excuses are what people use to feed fear. It rationalizes failures to comfort emotions. I hear people say "I do not have enough time to work out," or "I have tried everything and nothing works." Realistically, all I hear them saying is "sacrificing time for something they do not think they can conquer is not worth working for," or that they have attempted something and failed at it one time more than they anticipated that they would. Simply put, it is all just excuses.

There are millions of excuses so it is easy for someone to use them to convey why they are not fit instead of trying to change their attitude. When you have to use excuses to justify your decision-making process to yourself, you know you need some help. I cannot imagine someone not having enough time to do anything.

Everyone on earth has the same 168 hours in a week, so not having enough time is like not having enough air to breathe. STOP making excuses. Fix the problem instead of running from it. If time is the factor that is limiting you from reaching your goals, analyze your schedule and figure out how many "free" hours you can afford to invest into your goal each weak. Add up all the hours you spend cooking, working, shopping, sleeping, cleaning, and whatever else you do each week and minus if from 168. That would let you know how much possible time you have to devote your energy towards your goal. GET UP and GO!

The people who fall victim to failure and use excuses to supplement their emotions developed this behavior out of habit. The only way to change that behavior is to recognize the negative thought pattern you have embedded into yourself. You need to hold yourself accountable and reward yourself when you do recognize the negativity forming in your decision-making process.

Good habits take time to build. Think in terms of training your dog. When the dog disobeys your orders, they are punished. When the dog complies with your commands, they receive a treat. Hold yourself to the same standard. Incorporating small changes over a long period of time will develop better habits. Not only will identifying negative thinking patterns allow you to increase your positive re-enforcement in yourself, but it will allow you to capitalize on other people's weaknesses and fears of failure.

<u>MISERY LOVES COMPANY</u>

Naturally, peoples and their attitudes rub off on us. We as humans adapt to what is being thrown at us. If you're aspiring to reach a goal and keep receiving constant negativity, it can and probably will affect your performance. If you are attempting something that others have failed at, chances are that they will try to bring you down. I would not say that they are discouraging you intentionally but, their negativity will impede your success.

I have heard of people not even attempting their goal anymore because they fear everyone else being correct about them failing. They fear being a part of the statistics. Approach every situation with a positive attitude. If you put in the work, you will reap the benefits the lifestyle has to offer you. How can someone who failed then tell you that you will not succeed? Do not cater advice from these types of people. Instead, speak to those who succeeded.

I would not find it wise to take advice from a broke person on how to get rich, nor would I ask someone who is lost for directions. Surrounding yourself with people who inspire you to do better, people with the same goal as you, and with people who have already accomplished the goal you are trying to reach will propel you closer to success. Attitudes are contagious. Success is the result of time and effort combined. There are no shortcuts. Conquering failures in fitness builds psychological strength and confidence in every aspect of life. Once you learn to control your attitude, you will effectively guide your decision-making process without the use of emotions.

UPDATE FROM THE AUTHOR'S DRIVE

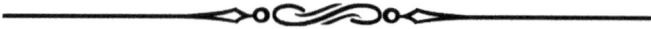

During the drafting of this book, I was undergoing my appeals for the charges that I stand convicted of. Along the journey, I had sleepless nights reading my record of trial and studying the law, enough to rectify my wrongful conviction. After almost 2 ½ years of working with my attorney to plea my case, the appellant court overturned the sentence part of my conviction and lowered my twenty-five-year sentence by a decade.

As this book is still being written, I am still fighting my conviction. I say all that to say this; Progress is a form of elevation. The results you want will not come easy but they will come eventually. Everything takes time. As we get ready to attack the physical challenges in this book, just remember that *everything takes time*. Keep on working and you will reap the fruits of your labor. Keep pushing.

"Go as far as you can see and when you get there you would be able to see further," Thomas Carlyle.

PART III

PHYSICAL

"The purpose of training is to tighten up the slack, toughen up the body, and to polish the spirit," Morihei Ueshiba.

CHAPTER 6

GOAL IDENTIFICATION

"The most recognized part of fitness is the *physical* aesthetics of one's body. The body is the display of the results you get from mastering both the *mental* and *emotional* parts of the lifestyle. This section will help assist you in identifying your physical fitness goal which in turn will help direct you to the best approach in order to reach that goal."

PHYSICAL ATTRIBUTE

Through consistency, hard work, and perseverance, a fit body becomes the icon of disciplined behavior. A fit body is symbolic of good health as well as good habits. There are many approaches to obtaining the trophy of fitness but first, you will have to take into consideration that everyone's body is different, so physically, everyone's fitness goal may be similar but never the same.

Some people may want to lose weight while others may want to gain muscle. The most important part of the process is distinguishing between both what it is you want physically and identifying the best approach to reaching that goal. A goal physically can be as simple as wanting abs or as complex as losing 200 pounds. Both are attainable goals but require two completely different approaches. It is critical that you select the proper method to help you reach your goal specifics.

"You can't hop on a plane to New York City and expect to land in Los Angeles."

YOU ARE YOUR BIGGEST CRITIC

Before determining what your goal is specifically, keep in mind when setting a personal goal that you do not want to be the judge of yourself. You are your biggest critic. You look at yourself every day whether through a mirror, a picture, or even the shower. The slight difference that your body may undergo may not be something that you yourself may notice which can be discouraging.

This is because you have seen the entire evolution. Day by day. Do you notice when your hair grows longer? How about your nails? No. But eventually, it gets to a point where the difference becomes noticeable. It is no different from seeing a friend you have not seen in quite some time. When you finally see this person, any small changes that may have occurred to their appearance is forefront. You notice the smallest changes because to you, these changes took effect over the course of your separation.

The body translates its changes in the same manner. The change occurs ever so slightly that the naked eye may not recognize it immediately. This is why it is necessary to set a goal, formulate a plan to reach that goal, and use checkpoints along the way to track your development and progress. As discussed in Chapter 1, your motivator is a key element in establishing a strong motivation. Using stepping stones to position you closer to the final destination.

"Go as far as you can see. When you get there, you will be able to see further,"
Thomas Carlyle.

Focus on completing your goal while you embrace the process that comes with it.

GOAL IDENTIFICATION

In order for a desire to meet the requirements of a goal, it has to be well-defined. The goal has to be realistic and achievable or else it will just be a fantasy.

STEPS FOR IDENTIFYING A GOAL

When setting a physical goal, you need to be specific in your desires. This requires you to take time and reflect on exactly what it is you are looking for. Identifying your goal will prevent you from walking around the gym, aimlessly picking workouts that do not correlate with what you are trying to achieve. If you work your ass off doing all the wrong things, you will end up somewhere you do not want to be. So again, your goal should contain detailed information. It is easy to say "I want to lose weight." I'm sure you do! But, what is your goal? 10lbs? 20lbs? 100lbs? Losing weight is a blanket statement and leaves too much room for interpretation. It does not provide you with a goal to push towards. A more direct statement would be "I want to lose 40lbs." Automatically, you can create a physical finish line. The direct approach allows you to see that your goal is tangible.

After identifying your goal, you will need to test yourself to find out your current status in relation to your objective. If your goal is to run a six-minute mile, find out how long it currently takes you to complete a mile run. If your goal is to lose 40 lbs, weigh yourself in your current state. Figuring out where you currently are in comparison to your goal will allow you to track and measure your progression and performance along the journey. This track record will give you some insight as to if the training program you have selected is an efficient learning opportunity for adjustments.

Now that you have a goal and know how far away from that goal you are, you will be able to set a realistic deadline by which you are to reach your goal by. This date will keep you ambitious, allowing you to challenge yourself not to fall short of a specific time period or be susceptible to procrastination.

EXAMPLES OF GOALS

WHAT IS NOT A GOAL	HOW A GOAL SHOULD LOOK
I want to lose weight.	I want to lose 40lbs by _____ *(Insert Date)* I currently weigh _____lbs Today is _____ *(Insert Date)*
I want to get stronger.	I want to bench press _____lbs by _____ *(Insert Date)* My current max is _____ *(Insert Max)* Today is _____
I want to run faster.	I want to run a mile under ____ minutes by _____ *(Insert Date)* It currently takes me __ minutes and __ seconds. Today is _____
My goal is	

By this step, your goal should be properly formatted in terms of what it is that you want, where and how far you are away from it, and when you want it by. This will put you through the complex process of finding a form of fitness you would like to practice. What makes this process difficult is the research that may be needed to identify what each style entails.

There is a variety of fitness styles, each being similar in nature but differs in practice. Look at it like karate. You have many styles such as Ju-Jit-Su, Shotokan, Ma-Tai, etc. Each style may teach you how to defend yourself or strike a proper attack, but none are taught the same way.

TYPES OF FITNESS STYLES

Bodybuilding-This type of fitness style relies primarily on weight training to sculpt the body into its most possible aesthetic structure. This form isolates muscle groups so that they are targeted individually to capitalize on muscle development. This book is designated to this training style.

Cross Fit-This type of fitness focuses on mobility, catering to those who enjoy a high-intensity training exercise program. This form incorporates body weight exercises, ropes, bands, kettle bells, and weights, not really making muscular development the primary focus but instead, muscle endurance.

Power lifting-This form of fitness is exactly what it sounds like. People who practice this form are trying to become as strong as possible. This style of fitness requires you to lift heavy weights, usually for low repetitions to capitalize on strength development.

Yoga-This form of fitness focuses primarily on stretching and breathing techniques to loosen and contract the muscles. This form will help increase your flexibility and provide the body with opportunities to promote proper blood flow.

If you're asking yourself if you have to pick only one style, the answer is NO.

General Fitness-This form is the standard fitness approach and incorporates a little bit of multiple styles into one. This style allows for flexibility in programs to accommodate for specific physical needs.

Essentially, your goal helps decide which form or style is best for you to practice. It is not a bad idea to add bits and pieces from multiple styles as long as it contributes to the overall goal instead of taking away from it. In fact, it may be best to do so in order to identify which style it is you like best.

Before you go to the next chapter, take a look at your goal again. If you can find a picture of someone you idolize who has already reached your physical goal, take a look at it. Remember this picture because this will help you when it is all over. **HARD WORK PAYS OFF!**

CHAPTER 7

EATING HABITS

———————————⇒∘⟨⟩∘⇐———————————

A majority of the results that derives from the rigorous physical training are reflected from proper eating habits. It is such discipline which separates the ability to reach a specific goal from not reaching it. Nutrition serves as approximately 50% if not more of the "work" needed to attain a physical goal.

We've all heard someone say the words *"I need to go on a diet"* before. The conception of the word diet has an implication of eating healthy but in reality, the two differs significantly. Dieting consists of limiting someone eating capabilities and quantities by omitting certain foods from consumption. Eating healthy on the other hand is simply making better selections based on nutritional value. Companies have capitalized on the ignorance of human beings by accommodating their agenda of *"dieting"* by promoting low fat foods. They advertise their products with a special reduced sugars, fats and/or salts encouraging people to indulge in their already established eating habits. Companies have even taken it a step further by boldly advertising their bottles with calorie counts to comfort the customers further extending their tactics. Labelling products "more clearly" does not fix the problem of making people choose better alternatives. Soda is soda regardless of the calorie count or reduced sugars. It is still an acidic drink which is unhealthy and would remain to be known as one of the main contributions towards obesity.

With fitness, it is necessary to recognize these disguises and use them to your own advantage. What good is any knowledge on a problem if you are going to let the problem manifest and do you harm anyway. When considering eating habits, it is best to recognize that there are always better alternatives. Personally, I gave up eating fast food in the year 2016 as one of my New Year resolutions. However, for example purposes, I will pick on McDonalds. Certain diets would prevent someone from consuming McDonalds entirely. The habit of eating healthy would only encourage better decision making of the meal you select. Human nature says when constantly subjecting yourself to battle temptation, temptation wins. God gave us the freedom of choice and so when you take the ability to make a choice away from a person, they will feel as if they are losing control of a situation. You make a choice every time you are getting ready to order a meal. Instead of ordering that sloppy triple cheese burger with fries and a soda, take into account that grilled chicken sandwich or grilled chicken salad that is right next to it on the menu. If you like drinking carbonated drinks, instead of soda consider flavored sparkling water. Get acclimated with the better choices that are available to you. Going out and eating like trash expecting great results in the gym is crazy. That is being an oxymoron. It is like winding down the windows in a vehicle and turning on the A.C because you are hot. Counterproductive.

As I mentioned previously, something has to be excluded for the program you are on to be considered a diet. Usually, when you hear someone bring up being on a diet, they tell you everything that they cannot have as oppose to what they look forward to having. Let's face it, dieting sounds miserable. Limiting people's options is the best way to make them give up. To elaborate a little more an example of a diet is the Ketogenic diet. The "Keto" diet for those who don't know is a diet that is increasing in popularity due to the results of weight loss people have been claiming to see from it. Does it work? Yes. But is it painful? Absolutely! The diet consists of low carbs and high fat foods which forces the body into a state known as ketosis. While your body is undergoing ketosis instead of burning carbs for energy, it uses fat. Ideally, this diet is not one I would recommend to someone who lacks discipline because so much is being sacrificed. Foods such as bread, pasta, rice and potatoes would go against the diet. Not everyone has the proper mindset to attack the diet with 100% commitment. Once a person breaks a diet once, they will lose motivation to continue because they would feel as if they have already failed taking one step back. Furthermore, diets are only temporary. It is almost as probative as putting yourself on a budget. It is hard to control unforeseeable circumstances in life so by practicing proper habits, it alleviates the headache of the unknown. Allowing yourself to have proper saving/spending habits will prevent you from having to budget in the midst of an emergency. Having good eating habits consistently prevents you from having to starve yourself to drop 10 pounds because your vacation is coming up or summer is around the corner. Control the aspects of your life that are controllable. Remember, failure is a loss and there is no losses in fitness, but only lessons.

When eating healthy you have a variety of nutritious foods that helps the body function better. Protein filled foods such as fish, chicken, turkey, beef, beans, etc., helps with muscle growth and recovery. Think of it in terms of the muscle is "broken down" through exercise, protein *fills into the cracks of the breakdown of the muscle* and the tissue the muscle grows during the during the recovery stage grows over the "protein and muscle breakdown" making the muscle grow in size. Vegetables and fruits, such as beets, avocados and asparagus help burn fat. You may also find proper nutrition through other greens, such as spinach and kale. What you consume determines how the body performs and transform. What people fail to realize is that not all the time you have to consume meat for the source of protein. Look at some of the biggest animals in the jungle. A gorilla, elephant, even giraffe, none of them consume meat but they are all huge. When it comes to eating healthier in the fitness game, look at it as the rule of substitution. If someone in the NBA is not performing well, the coach calls a timeout and make substitutions and adjustments necessary to win the game. The same applies here. There is always an alternative to cleaner eating. Instead of white bread, eat wheat. Instead of soda, drink juice. Instead of white rice, try brown rice. Instead of chip ahoy cookies, eat oatmeal and peanuts. If you insist on having a cookie, don't go for Oreos when the oatmeal raisin cookies are right across from it. Healthier alternatives go a long way over the course of time.

Monitoring what you eat can get you to your results faster. If you have a calorie surplus, you will gain weight. If you have a calorie deficit, you will lose weight. You must already realize that the time you consume these calories matter as well. Eating before you sleep will allow sugars to stick to your body fat, because your body will not be expending energy to burn off the calories. Also, foods containing tryptophan, which boost melatonin, a sleeping aid that the body produces, makes good pre-bed-time snacks. Some of these foods will be yogurt, almonds, fish or poultry.

I will give you only guidelines to help assist you with your fitness venture. Again, these are only guidelines because I cannot restrict you to a specific diet without proper consultation.

NOTE: The next 3 examples are for a person consuming 3000 calories daily

Maintaining

Maintaining means that you are not really trying to gain weight nor lose weight. You are content with where you are and just trying to remain consistent with what it is you already got. I use maintenance phase to transition in or out of a bulk phase to or from a shred phase. It can constitute as a good medium to ensure a smooth transition.

You should be consuming roughly 14-16 calories per body weight daily/

30% of your calories should be protein (roughly 1g of protein per body weight), 45% of your calories should be carbs (roughly 1.5g-1.7g per body weight) and 25% of your calories should be fats (roughly 0.4g per body weight).

Divide by 4 for protein- Divide by 4 for carbs- Divide by 9 for fats

In context if you are consuming 3000 calories a day multiply it by the percent you are trying to calculate and that will tell you how much to consume.

EXAMPLE:

3000 calories x .30 (protein) = 900 / 4 = 225g protein per day
3000 calories x .45 (carbs) = 1350 / 4 = 337.5g carbs per day
3000 calories x .25 (fats) = 750 / 9 = 83.3 g fats per day

Shredding

During this phase, you are trying to burn body fat but still retain the muscle that you have. To lose weight, you need to have a calorie deficit or expend a lot of the calories that you are taking in. I would advise to drop your calories roughly 25% when shredding, because too much of a drop will make you lose weight too fast and not have the finished look that you may be going for. Typically, you should be in this phase for roughly 12 weeks.

You should be consuming roughly 10-12 calories per body weight daily.

40% of your calories should be protein (roughly 1.1g of protein per body weight), 40% of your calories should be carbs (roughly 1.1g per body weight) and 20% of your calories should be fats (roughly 0.25g per body weight).

Divide by 4 for protein- Divide by 4 for carbs- Divide by 9 for fats
3000 calories x .40 (protein) = 1200 / 4 = 300 g protein per day
3000 calories x .40 (carbs) = 1200 / 4 = 300g carbs per day
3000 calories x .20 (fats) = 600 / 9 = 66.6 g fats per day

Bulking

During this phase, you are trying to add muscle. This would require you to have a caloric surplus. You also need to retain most of the calories you are taking in rather than expending, so you should reduce your cardio. Overeating and increasing calorie intake may sound the same in nature, but they both differ. Overeating will lead to stretching your stomach lining and increasing your fat stores, which is not the goal here. Your insulin level will drop, which is contradictory to what we are trying to achieve. Your insulin controls fat resistance and muscle building. Instead of overeating in one sitting, break your meals down into smaller portions and eat them throughout the day until your nutritional goal is met. Typically, you should be in this phase for 12-16 weeks.

You should be consuming roughly 10-12 calories per body weight daily.

30% of your calories should be protein (roughly 1.2g of protein per body weight), 50% of your calories should be carbs (roughly 2.1g per body weight) and 20% of your calories should be fats (roughly 0.35g per body weight).

Divide by 4 for protein- Divide by 4 for carbs- Divide by 9 for fats
3000 calories x .30 (protein) = 900 / 4 = 225 g protein per day
3000 calories x .50 (carbs) = 1500 / 4 = 375g carbs per day
3000 calories x .20 (fats) = 600 / 9 = 66.6 g fats per day

CHAPTER 8

GENERAL UNDERSTANDING OF BODY BUILDING

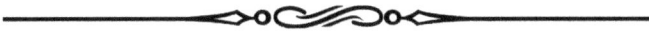

BODYBUILDING

Some hear the word bodybuilding and just think BIG. Bodybuilding is a science that has been around since the 1940s. The primary focus is to get the best physique, development, symmetry, and definition a bodybuilder can make their body attain. This is done by intensely training each muscle group with weights that take advantage of different angles using different exercises and equipment.

Incorporated with these exercises is the acknowledgment and science of nutrition. The development of each muscle is determined by the clarity of the muscles. Bodybuilding and its principles not only help with mental health, physical health, sexual health, and your psychological well-being, but it also provides one of the best aesthetic outcomes for your body physically. Bodybuilding, with its techniques and principles, can be used for training anyone and is able to help almost anyone as well. **LET'S DIG IN.**

Going into bodybuilding, you need a solid foundation because there will be times when the weight is physically challenging, but your mental state will determine the execution of the lift. It is the body that follows the mind. Failure does not exist in the bodybuilding world because every attempt alone makes you stronger.

IDENTIFYING KEY PARTS OF THE BODY

There are over 500 muscles in the body. However, in bodybuilding, we focus on a few specific muscle groups. Bodybuilding relies primarily on weight training to sculpt the body into its most aesthetic structural build. This form of fitness isolates muscle groups so that they are targeted individually to capitalize on each muscle development. These groups, in part are:

CHEST
BACK
SHOULDERS
LEGS
ARMS
ABS

Each of these muscle groups contains subdivisions that allow us to intricately target the overall muscle in focus from every angle. A general idea of this would be:

CHEST	**Back**	**Shoulders**
Upper Pectoral Lower pectoral Mid Chest Cavity	Latissimus Dorsi (referred to as LATS) Spinal Erectors (Lower) Mid Back	Front Deltoids (Referred to as DELTS) Side Deltoids Rear Deltoids Trapezius (Referred to as TRAPS)

Legs	Arms	Abs
Quadriceps (Referred to as QUADS)	Biceps	Upper Abdomen
Hamstrings	Triceps	Lower Abdomen
Calves	Forearms	Mid Abdomen
		Obliques
NOTE:	NOTE: The Bicep is composed of 2 Heads.	
Quadriceps have 4 heads	Long Head (Outer)	
Vastus Lateralis	Short Head (Inner)	
Vastus Medialis	NOTE: The Tricep is composed of 3 Heads.	
Vastus Intermedius	Lateral Head	
Rectus Femoris	Long Head	
	Medial Head	

Understanding the muscle and its composition is important because aesthetically, everyone is different. Some people may have been gifted with a genetic build that is better than others. Learning how to identify and target a particular muscle allows opportunities for thickness and definitions to any area needed. Starting off, you will need to learn the basic lifts to help build strength and conditioning in order to be effective during your program. As you progress, you can implement different techniques listed in this book to intensify your workout. Each muscle group has "basic" lifts that will be necessary but not mandatory to build a solid foundation. Some of these workouts would generally be:

CHEST	BACK
Bench Press (Flat, Incline, and Decline) Dumbell Press (Flat, Incline, and Decline) Flys Push Ups	Deadlifts Rows (Barbell and Dumbbell) Pull Downs Pull Ups
SHOULDERS	**LEGS**
Military Press (Overhead) Arnold Press Raises (Lateral and Front)	Squat Leg Press Leg Extensions (Quads) Leg Curl (Hamstrings) Lunges

ARMS (BICEPS)	ARMS (TRICEPS)	ABS
Dumbbell Curls E-Z Bar Curl Barbell Curl	Close-grip Bench Press Tricep Extensions Skull Crushers	Crunches Leg Raises Planks

ACTIVATION OF THE MUSCLE

Each lift that is done has a particular muscle in which is the primary target. Many movements, however, require other muscles to take secondary effects to assist in lifting the weight. A Mind-Muscle connection is needed to assure that you are using the muscle intended to be targeted. This is the mental aspect of each lift which makes sure you are providing contractions to the primary focus. For example, the bench press. When on the bench press, the primary muscle is the chest. Assuming that your intended focus is the chest, the bar should be held at shoulder width or wider to assure that the chest is being activated when the movement is being conducted. In the same instance, the triceps are being activated to help with the lift. This muscle automatically becomes secondary due to the lift being a pressing movement.

Any movement that involves a "pulling" motion incorporates the Biceps.

Any movement that involves a "pushing" motion incorporates the Triceps.

Dumbbell movements work the stabilizer muscles.

UNDERSTANDING PROGRAM DEVELOPMENTS

Looking at your workout plan, you may just choose an exercise on the "to-do" list and get it done in any order of your liking. However, the building of a workout plan and the order of your exercises should compliment the goal that you are trying to reach.

A majority of workout plans (at least the good ones) that focus on size and strength make sure that your compound movements and exercises are done first. These are the exercises that require you to use two or more joints and are usually done using a barbell or a machine that requires you to load weight on it (i.e., LEG PRESS). Usually, this is the heaviest lift of the exercises on that "to-do" list. Doing them first prevents you from suffering from muscle fatigue which would be a problem if you were to try to do it further into the workout. Not only will you be tired and compromise the effectiveness of your workout, but it will also effect the amount of weight you can lift which makes you more susceptible to injury. Form is always compromised when the weight becomes too heavy.

Post-compound lifts, free weights are usually next on the agenda. Free weights consist of dumbbells, kettlebells, weighted balls, etc. This equipment allows you the freedom of movement and also extends the range of motion beyond what is possible with your compound lifts. Free weights like your compound movements, encompass mass and strength. However, free weights work on your stabilizer muscles as well.

Lastly, machines and cables are done towards the end of the workouts for isolation and strategic development. Machines, unlike your compound movements and free weights, are tailored to a specific pathway, with every repetition allowing you to focus primarily on the muscle at hand. This becomes an advantage later on in your intermediate/advanced bodybuilding stages.

SETS

When preparing a workout plan, one of the major considerations to take into account is the number of sets needed to be performed per muscle group, per exercise, and per workout. A SET is a group of completed repetitions that is divided by a rest period. This is one of the contributing factors that effects the total volume that a muscle will endure (Sets x Reps=Volume). Finding the right amount that aligns with your goal is essential because too many sets will lead to over-training while too little will make you leave gains on the table and we are not trying to do that.

Typically, a general idea for body building is 3-6 sets per exercise with 4 being ideal; (this is in relation to the total number of exercises that you plan on doing for that muscle group). A whole workout should consist of roughly 10-24 working sets. Your warm-up sets are not considered to be a working set. If more than one muscle group is being trained in the same workout session, the number of sets for the entirety of the workout session should never pass 40. Exceeding 40 may hinder muscle growth and recovery and again when exhaustion is a factor, cause injury.

REPS

Another consideration for the preparation of a workout plan is the number of repetitions (reps) needed per exercise. A **REP** is a completed rotation of the combination of the concentric (lift motion) and eccentric (lowering motion) parts of a lift. Think of a rep as how many times you can REPeat the action at task. The contraction and extension collectively make a rep. Multiple reps collectively equal a set. The number of reps needed per exercise varies per goal as well. The heavier the weight, the fewer amounts of reps you are going to be able to do, and vice versa. The lighter the weight, the more reps you will be able to do.

As a guideline for beginners and intermediate-level bodybuilders, it is recommended to use typically 70-75% of your **1 Rep Maximum** (1RM) to build both strength and mass. This will allow you to complete roughly 6-12 reps for the upper body and 10-16 reps for the lower body for multiple sets. To reiterate, this is just a guideline but until you are certain of your goal and the route you need to take to get there, this will be the safest approach to increasing muscle growth and overall strength. Altering the weight would require you to assess the entire workout plan to ensure the reps and sets correlate with the projected goal.

REP GUIDELINE

STRENGTH	4-6
MUSCLE HYPERTROPHY	8-12
MUSCLE ENDURANCE	12 and above

1 REP MAXIMUM (1RM)

Your 1RM is the maximum amount of weight you can lift successfully one time for a full repetition. This number is a measurement used to gauge total strength with an exercise and is usually tested on the bench press, squat rack, and dead lift. All of your lifts should be calculated in relation to your 1RM.

WEIGHT IN RELATION TO YOUR 1RM

	WEIGHT
20 REPS	**45% OF YOUR 1RM**
15 REPS	**55% OF YOUR 1RM**
12 REPS	**65% OF YOUR 1RM**

10 REPS	75% OF YOUR 1RM
8 REPS	80% OF YOUR 1RM
6 REPS	85% OF YOUR 1RM
4 REPS	90% OF YOUR 1RM
2 REPS	95% OF YOUR 1RM
1 REP	100% = YOUR 1RM

To calculate a percentage of your 1RM, you can use the formula below:

MAX WEIGHT X PERCENTAGE = THE DESIGNATED PERCENTAGE OF YOUR 1 REP MAX

Example: Let's say your dead lift max is 500lbs and you want to do working sets of 10. You will input into a calculator **500 x .75 = 375.**

500 would be your max weight, .75 is the percentage in relation to your max according to the chart and 375 becomes 75% of your max weight which is what you should be using to complete your working sets of 10 reps. As a general rule of thumb, when completing your reps, you want to use weight in which when you hit the total amount of reps you are targeting, you are at the point of reaching muscle failure.

So, if the goal is to get 10 reps and by the time you reach 10 reps you feel as if you could have done any more reps, you should go up in weight to capitalize on your gains. To ensure you are getting a bang for your buck, by the time you reach roughly 8 out of your 10 reps, you should feel as if you may not make it to 10 but of course, strive and complete the set. This would be one of the advantages of having a spotter, which is someone who can assist you with the lift in the event that you are unable to get it yourself.

The most effective rep range for gaining muscle mass is 8-12 reps. As far as shredding and losing body fat, the best approach would be the 12-15 rep range. This may even be extended upwards towards 20 reps depending on the exercise.

CALCULATING YOUR 1 REP MAXIMUM

Some programs are based off of your max numbers. It is always good to know roughly where you stand in regard to your maximum lifts. The best way to calculate your 1RM is to actually get under some heavy weight and just lift it until you physically can not lift anymore. There is nothing more motivational in the gym than throwing around heavy weights, or setting a new personal record (**PR**). This will be the most natural way to conduct this measurement. However, there is a secondary option using a formula that provides you with an estimated max using the number of reps you can complete with the weight you used. This is known as the *EPLEY FORMULA*.

The formula is:

1RM = {1+(0.0333 x number of reps completed)} x weight lifted

So, if maxed out at 15 reps with 315 on dead lifts, the formula would look like this.

1RM = {1 + (0.333 x 15)} x 315

1RM = 1.4995 x 315

1RM = 472.34lbs (Rough Estimate)

TRAINING SPLIT

The way your workouts are divided by the days of the week is known as a training split. Each training split varies per goal and the number of times you exercise weekly with the number of times you decide to target a specific muscle group weekly. As a beginner/intermediate-level bodybuilder, you would want a split that allows you to target a majority of muscle groups per workout session. Building a strong foundation is essential and though the split alone does not ensure maximum growth, it has an influence on the totality of every workout necessary for that growth. When picking a split, pick one that is convenient to your work-out schedule and the days that you can get into the gym.

There are 3-day splits that allow muscles to be worked 2 times a week.

There are 4-day splits which allow an additional day in which you can use for spot training to target weak points.

There are 5-day splits that allow you to exercise each muscle group individually.

Choosing a split depends on several factors such as training experience, goals, convenience, schedule, and the number of times you can work out a week. When creating a split, do not group two muscle groups back to back which requires the same secondary muscle. For example, the chest and shoulder both shares the triceps as a secondary muscle. It would be a good idea to separate those two days to ensure your triceps can get enough recovery time to do what they actually need to do when the day comes for you to put it to work.

Training splits for beginners:

MON	TUE	WED	THUR	FRI	SAT	SUN
PUSH	PULL	LEGS	OFF	PUSH	PULL	LEGS

Push refers to pressing exercises which primarily involve the use of shoulders chest and triceps.

Pull refers to pulling exercises that primarily would involve the use of the back and biceps.

Legs, of course, refer to leg exercises.

Though this training split has picked up heavily in the bodybuilding world more recently, I will recommend this split for beginners. The reason being is that this program allows you to work each muscle group twice a week where you can separate your compound lifts from your static lifts. This advantage of exercising a muscle group allows room to tailor a program necessary to bulk or shred by allowing each muscle group to endure a higher volume of work per week.

MON	TUE	WED	THUR	FRI	SAT	SUN
CHEST AND TRICEPS	BACK AND BICEPS	OFF	SHOUL-DERS	ARMS	LEGS	OFF

This training split allows you to group muscle groups that have a secondary effect on the primary muscle. For example, as you do chest, you are incorporating your triceps to "press" the bar up. Because the triceps are already being activated, it may serve as an advantage to "double tap" them with isolated exercises. If you plan to do a split like this, you must be sure not to exhaust the secondary muscle before the primary has a chance to get fatigued.

The advantage in this split is that it also allows you to target your arms twice a week as opposed to once, making you access muscle fibers that have not been reached earlier in the week. This split is designed for someone who goes to the gym 5 days a week.

__MON__	__TUE__	__WED__	__THUR__	__FRI__	__SAT__	__SUN__
UPPER BODY	LOWER BODY	OFF	UPPER BODY	LOWER BODY	OFF	REPEAT

Upper body refers to the chest, back, shoulders, and arms
The lower body refers to legs and abs.

This split has many advantages for beginners. It allows adequate rest after 2 workout sessions which is vital for recovery. This split also promotes a larger volume for each muscle group due to each group being targeted nearly 3 times a week.

__Advanced training splits:__

MON	TUE	WED	THUR	FRI	SAT	SUN
CHEST	BACK	SHOULDER	OFF	ARMS	LEGS	REPEAT/ OFF

This split isolates every muscle group per day allowing you to focus on the muscle at hand. The extra attention that the muscle group will be getting will allow you to specifically target the muscle from every angle possible while all the other muscle groups get to rest and recover. The advantage of this split is that any parts falling behind can get undivided attention during the day of that muscle group. This split is designed for

5-6 days training split depending on how many off days you would like to permit.

MON	TUE	WED	THUR	FRI	SAT	SUN
CHEST MAJOR	BACK MAJOR	SHOUL-DER MAJOR	LEG MAJOR	ARMS MAJOR	OFF	RE-PEAT
BACK MINOR	SHOUL-DER MINOR	LEG MINOR	ARM MINOR	CHEST MINOR	OFF	RE-PEAT

This is one of my favorite splits. It allows you to activate a muscle group 1 day prior to heavy training of that muscle. With this split, you capitalize on gains as if you did the same muscle group two times in one day except the training is divided by a good night's sleep. Also, I've noticed with this training, that this actually helps warm up my muscles a little better in anticipation of the "real deal".

On major days, that muscle group is primary. This means that all the heavy lifts should be done on this day. For example, on leg major day, you should complete your squats, straight leg deadlifts, leg presses, or any heavy movements you will normally conduct on this leg day.

The minor on each day means this muscle group is secondary. This means only the static lifts should be conducted and you should be lifting moderate light for a numerous amount of reps. For example, on leg minor day, you should be completing your leg extensions, leg curls, calve raises, etc.

FULL RANGE OF MOTION

During an exercise, the complete expansion and extension following a contraction is the proper way to complete a repetition. This will ensure that every muscle fiber in the entire muscle is being activated and used to assist during a lift. The full expansion allows the muscle to stretch and expand and anything stretched out is always bigger than its condensed version. Doing half repetitions will risk leaving muscle fibers untouched, essentially leaving up to 50% of the muscle unaccounted for. The fear of not completing a lift is usually what drives someone to develop this bad behavior. For the best and fastest results, ensure yourself that you are completing the full range of motion on every lift.

45LB BARBELL PYRAMID SCHEME

During certain exercises, the increase of weight is usually done methodically. Too big of an increase can lead to an injury while too small of an increase can allow you to not capitalize on your workout. The proper increase depends on how many sets you have for the exercise and how many reps you have to conduct in total per exercise. As you would learn through experience, choosing the right amount of weight is crucial to ensure you are not only doing the exercises correctly but to make sure you are hitting your muscle hypertrophy point as well for muscle growth. These increases are usually what you would see in a gym using a barbell.

20 LB INCREASE	50 LB INCREASE THEN 20+ LB INCREASE	90 LB INCREASE
135	135	135
155	185	225
175	205	315
195	225	405
215	245	495
235	275	585
255	295	675
275	315	
295		

NOTE: In the event you cannot add the recommended amount, add less or stay at the same weight.

GRIPS WITH A BARBELL

Depending on the exercise, the barbell may be held in different grips to assist you with the lift or to increase the intensity of a lift. There are three different ways to grip a barbell:

Overhand grip which is standard. This is when your backhand is facing toward you. This is typically done on a bench press.

Underhand grip which is when your palms are facing toward you. This is typically done during rowing exercises or curls with the barbell.

Mixed grip which is when you have one hand in the overhand grip and the other is in an underhand grip. This is typically done with deadlifts and heavy barbell shrugs.

CHAPTER 9

SHOULDERS

———⊸o⌒⌒o⊶———

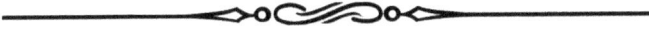

FRONT DELTOIDS

SIDE DELTOIDS

REAR DELTOIDS

TRAPEZIUS

COMPOSITION OF THE SHOULDERS

The separation of the shoulders refers to the deltoid also known as delts, found in the upper area of the arm. Their composition consists of three heads which are the anterior deltoid which is located in the front, the middle deltoid, and the posterior deltoid which is the rear head. The deltoid begins at the clavicle and the scapula and extends to the upper arm. The trapezius muscle is technically part of the shoulders, as it supports the back muscles because of its position between the shoulder blades.

ACTIVATION OF THE MUSCLE

Activation of the muscle usually includes but is not limited to lateral movements or presses above the head.

Front Deltoid Exercises- Arnold presses, military presses, front dumbbell raises.

Side Deltoid Exercises- Dumbbell lateral raises

Rear Deltoid Exercises- Bent-over lateral raises, incline bench laterals

Trapezius (TRAPS) Exercises- Barbell shrugs, dumbbell shrugs, clean and presses, upright rows.

SHOULDER EXERCISES

ARNOLD PRESSES

Primary Purpose: Front and Side Deltoids
Secondary Purpose: Triceps
Function: Seated on a 90-degree chair, place one dumbbell in each hand with elbows in front of you, and palms facing towards you.

Movement: Press the Dumbbell over your head, rotating your hands so that your palms are outwards at the top of the movement. (2) Lower the weight, rotating your wrist back to the starting position.

Note: Do not fully extend your arms. This will help maintain stress in your deltoids.

MILITARY PRESS

Primary purpose: Front and side deltoids
Secondary Purpose: Triceps
Function: Standing or seated, grip a barbell with an overhand grip, slightly outside of shoulder width, and hold it above your head.

Movement: With the bar raised overhead (fully extended), lower the bar to chin level. (2) Press the bar back above your head to full extension.

Note: This movement is one of the few compound movements for shoulders in which you can go super heavy. Keep strict movement throughout the lift, emphasizing on shoulders more than the triceps.

DUMBELL SHOULDER PRESS (SEATED)

Primary Purpose: Front/Side Delts
Secondary Purpose: Triceps
Function: Seated on a bench with back support, hold a dumbbell in each hand with a neutral grip.
Movement: Bring the dumbbells to your shoulders with your palms facing outward. (2) Press the dumbbells simultaneously above the head until they touch one another than lower them back to the shoulder.
Note: This movement is similar to Arnold presses. However, you are able to lift heavier due to there being no rotation during the movement.

LATERAL RAISES

Primary Purpose: Side Deltoids
Secondary Purpose: Front and rear deltoids
Function: Hold a dumbbell in each hand with a neutral grip at your side.
Movement: Lift the weights simultaneously at your side, leading with your elbows as if you were a bird trying to flap its wings. (2) Slowly lower the weight back to the side of your body.
Note: Try to prevent yourself from swinging the weight by using momentum from the rocking torso or bending your knees.

FRONT DUMBBELL RAISES

Primary Purpose: Rear Deltoids
Secondary Purpose: Side Deltoids
Function: Stand up straight, holding a dumbbell in each hand with a neutral grip and palms facing each other.
Movement: Raise the weight to roughly eye level, turning the thumb downward while keeping a slight bend at the elbow. (2) Lower weight back down, controlled to starting position.

BENT OVER LATERALS (SEATED OR STANDING)

Primary purpose: Rear Deltoids
Secondary purpose: Side Deltoids

Function: Lean over 45 degrees holding a dumbbell in each hand with a neutral grip and palms facing each other.

Movement: Raise the weight to your side leading through the elbow while keeping a slight bend at the elbow. (2) Lower weight back down controlled to starting position.

REAR DELT RAISE (INCLINE BENCH)

Primary Purpose: Rear Deltoids

Function: Lean over 45 degrees holding a dumbbell in each hand with a neutral grip and palms facing each other.

Movement: Raise the weight to your side as if you are making the letter "T" keeping the elbow straight and leading with the pinky side of your hand. (2) Lower weight back down controlled to starting position.

DUMBBELL SHRUGS

Primary Purpose: Trapezius

Function: Stand with a dumbbell in each hand, at your side.

Movement: Raise your shoulders as high as you can, as if you are trying to make your shoulders touch your ears. (2) Hold the position for 1-2 seconds at the top and slowly return to starting position.

Note: You can go super heavy with this movement. Use pauses at the top of the rep to capitalize on fatiguing the muscle.

BARBELL SHRUGS

Primary Purpose: Trapezius

Secondary Purpose: Forearms

Function: Stand holding a barbell with an overhand grip or a mixed grip in front of your quadriceps.

Movement: Raise your shoulders as high as you can, as if you are trying to make your shoulders touch your ears. (2) Hold the position for 1-2 seconds at the top and slowly return to starting position.

Note: Using a barbell will allow you to add more weight as you are doing this movement as a compound lift. This exercise may also be done on the smith machine. (2) This exercise can be done using a trap bar which will allow you to hold the handles at your sides as opposed to in front of you.

UPRIGHT ROW

Primary Purpose: Trapezius
Secondary Purpose: Front
Function: Stand holding a barbell with an overhand grip with your hands placed inside shoulder length.
Movement: From the lower position, raise the bar, keeping your elbows pointing outward until the bar is under your chin. Contract your shoulders back to activate more of the trapezius muscles. (2) Lower the weight back to starting position.
Note: Try to keep your torso upright to avoid rocking. (2) This exercise can be done with an e-z bar as well, which I would actually recommend over the barbell.

SINGLE ARM DB PRESS

Primary Purpose: Side Deltoid/Traps
Secondary Purpose: Triceps
Function: Seated on a bench with back support, hold a dumbbell in each hand with a neutral grip.
Movement: Bring the dumbbells to your shoulders with your palms facing outward. (2) Press the dumbbells simultaneously above your head until they touch one another. (3) While the dumbbells are at the overhead position, press one side for the number of reps you are trying to complete. (4) When you finish one side, hold the other dumbbell above your head and complete the other side for the same amount of repetitions.
Note: The hold above the head allows you to stress your shoulder muscles a lot more than your average dumbbell presses.

CHAPTER 10

BACK

—⊶∘⫘⊷∘⊷—

LATTISIMUS DORSI

TRAPEZIUS

MID/UPPER BACK

SPINAL ERECTORS

LOWER BACK

COMPOSITION OF THE BACK

The back refers to the muscles to the rear of the torso. This reference includes the latissimus dorsi (also known as LATS) which is the largest muscle in the back; this muscle extends from under your shoulder (arm-pit area) to the lower part of the back on both sides of the body. Also included is the trapezius, which is an exterior extending from the neck to below the shoulder blades. The back also consists of spinal erectors which protect the nerve channels and keeps the spine erect. Lastly, are the rhomboids.

ACTIVATION OF THE MUSCLE

This muscle group is generally activated by pulling movements.

Full-back development- Deadlifts

Latissimus Dorsi (LAT) Exercises- Barbell rows, Lat-Pull Downs, One-Arm Dumbbell Rows, Pull-Ups, T-Bar Row.

Trapezius (TRAPS) Exercises- Barbell Shrugs, Dumbbell Shrugs, Clean and Presses, Upright Rows.

Mid/Upper-Back Exercises- Seated Rows, Barbell Rows (underhand and overhand).

Spinal erectors/Lower Back Exercises- Straight Leg Deadlifts, Good mornings.

BACK EXERCISES

DEADLIFTS

Primary Purpose: Full back development

Secondary Purpose: Legs, Traps, Glutes

Function: Place a barbell on the floor in front of you with the weight loaded for lift. Make sure your feet are roughly shoulder-width apart. (2) Bend down and grab the bar with a mixed grip (one overhand, the other underhand) keeping your chest and head up with your back straight.

Movement: Start the lift by using your legs to stand up, relieving the pressure off of your lower back. (2) As the bar crosses your knees, pull your shoulder blades back and continue to stand until you have stood all the way up. (3) Lower the weight back down by leaning slightly forward at the hips, bending your knees, and bringing the weight back down to ground level.

Note: Be sure not to spread your legs too far apart. Doing so will require you to incorporate your lower back which is one of the slowest recovering muscles in the body. (2) This exercise is a full-body workout and assists with overall strength and power development. (3) **DO NOT** round your back, as it may cause a spinal injury.

BARBELL ROW

Primary Purpose: Upper back
Secondary Purpose: Latissimus Dorsi (LATS)
Function: With your feet in a normal stance, place the barbell in front of your feet, grabbing the bar with an overhand or underhand grip outside of shoulder width.
Movement: Leaning forward roughly 45 degrees, keeping your torso straight and your knees slightly bent, pull the bar up until it makes contact with your body. (2) Lower the weight back down to a full extension.
Note: Underhand grip the bar should be brought to right around the belly button area. Overhand grip you should be able to lean further down to bring the bar closer to your chest. (2) Try to avoid rocking and swaying when bringing the bar up.

LAT-PULL DOWNS

Primary Purpose: Latissimus Dorsi (LATS)
Secondary Purpose: Biceps and Forearm flexors
Function: Sit upright facing the LAT pulldown machine with your knees secured under the pads provided. (2) Grab the straight bar or LAT bar with an overhand wide grip.
Movement: Pull the bar down to your chest squeezing your shoulder blades back. (2) Hold contraction from 1-2 seconds and then slowly control the weight back to the starting position getting a full stretch of the LATS.
Note: This movement can be done behind the neck which would give emphasis to the lower portion of the LATS a little more.

One-Arm Dumbbell Row

Primary Purpose: Latissimus Dorsi (LATS)
Secondary Purpose: Posterior Deltoid and slight Trapezius
Function: Using a bench for support, place one knee and hand that is on the same side of the body on the bench, leaving the opposite leg on the floor for support. Grab a dumbbell with a hand that is free.

Movement: Pull the dumbbell towards your side as high as possible as if you were trying to elbow someone behind you while keeping your torso straight (2) Lower the dumbbell back to full extension.

Note: It is crucial to concentrate on the back contraction and not just pull the weight using your arms.

PULL-UP

Primary Purpose: Latissimus Dorsi (LATS)
Secondary Purpose: Biceps and Mid Back
Function: Hang from a pull-up bar with an overhand grip outside of shoulder width.
Movement: Pull your body up towards the bar while trying to pull your shoulder blades back until your chin passes the bar. (2) Lower yourself back down to almost a full extension, keeping tension on your LATS throughout the movement.
Note: At the bottom of a rep, keeping a slight bend in the elbow would allow you to keep the back muscles engaged as opposed to a full extension, which would disengage the back for a short period of time until the next repetition is being performed. (2) Using the underhand grip changes the movement to a chin-up, emphasizing more on the biceps.

T-BAR ROW

Primary Purpose: Upper Back Thickness
Secondary Purpose: Latissimus Dorsi (LATS)
Function: Standing over a T-Bar, bend your knees slightly and lean forward roughly 45 degrees. (2) Grab the handles (or bar) with an overhand grip.
Movement: Pull the bar until the weights touch your chest. (2) Lower weight back down to full arm's length without touching the floor.
Note: Using smaller plates will allow you to get a slightly better range of motion during this movement. (2) Keep your back straight throughout the movement and avoid rocking or swaying as it will manipulate the contraction of the back.

SEATED ROW

Primary Purpose: Mid back/lower LATS
Secondary Purpose: Rear Deltoids and Biceps
Function: Sit on a row machine with your foot placed on the footrest. (2) With your knees bent and torso slightly bent forward, grab the handle of choice.

Movement: Pull the handle towards your sternum by pulling your elbows back and chest raised upright. (2) As the handle contacts your body, you should be sitting straight up with your shoulder blades pinched together. (3) Lower the weight back towards the rack in a controlled manner, emphasizing the contraction in your back.

Note: Try to prevent yourself from rounding your back or swaying back and forth when conducting your reps.

CHAPTER 11

CHEST

———⊷o⧼⧽o⊷———

UPPER PECTORAL

MID CHEST

LOWER PECTORAL

COMPOSITION OF THE CHEST

The separation of the chest consists of the upper pectoralis major which is attached to the collarbone. This portion is known as the clavicular portion. Secondly is the lower pectoralis major, which is known as the sternal portion. Exercises such as push-ups, dips, bench press, and dumbbell press ext., targets this muscle through its movements. Your pectorals sit on top of your rib cage. Holding a bar with a wide grip allows you to target the outside of the chest while holding the bar with a closer grip targets the inside portion of the chest.

ACTIVATION OF THE MUSCLE

Upper Pectoral Exercises – Incline Bench Press, Incline Dumbbell Press

Mid-Chest Exercises – Flat bench press, Flat dumbbell press, Single-arm dumbbell press, Push-ups, dumbbell flyes, cable flyes.

Lower Pectoral Exercises – Decline Bench Press, Decline Dumbbell Press

CHEST EXERCISES

Barbell Flat Bench Press

Primary Purpose: Mid-Chest

Secondary Purpose: Triceps and Front Deltoid slightly

Function: Lie on the bench and grip the bar outside of shoulder width, with an overhand neutral grip and feet planted on the floor. (2) Your back should have a natural arch to it and your LATS should be flared out.

Movement: Start the lift by un-racking the weight and holding it above your head at a full extension. (2) Lower the bar down until it contracts right below your sternum, keeping the elbows pointing outward. (3) After contact with the chest, raise the bar back up to the starting position, extending your arms fully.

Note: This exercise is the biggest compound movement for the chest and can be done at various angles (incline, decline, and flat). Incline capitalizes on the upper pectoral while decline capitalizes on the lower. (2) Try to use the heel of your foot, pushing against the floor to help you drive the weight back up.

Dumbbell Press

Primary Purpose: Mid/Outer Chest

Secondary Purpose: Triceps

Function: Lie down on a bench with a dumbbell in each hand. Hold the weight at full extension overhead with your palms facing outwards.

Movement: Lower the weights simultaneously as far as possible, making each dumbbell touch the outside of your pectorals. (2) Press the weight back up to starting position.

Note: You can make your palms face each other at the top of your repetition for a better contraction. (2) Dumbbells allow you to get a larger range of motion as opposed to barbells. Take advantage of this.

Dumbbell Flyes

Primary Purpose: Mid-Chest
Secondary Purpose: Front Deltoids
Function: Lie down on a bench with a dumbbell in each hand held above your head. Make sure your palms are facing each other and your elbows are slightly bent. Feet should be planted on the floor.
  Movement: Lower the weight to your side in a half-circle motion, extending as far as possible as if you were going to give someone a hug. (2) As you reach the bottom of the stretch, reverse the movement by raising the weight using the same half-circle motion you used to return back to the starting position.
  Note: Keep your arms bent slightly to prevent any elbow pain.

Barbell Incline Bench Press

Primary Purpose: Upper Chest
Secondary Purpose: Front Deltoids and Triceps
Function: Lie on an incline bench and grip the bar outside of shoulder width, with an overhand neutral grip and feet planted on the floor. (2) Your back should have a natural arch to it and your LATS should be flared out.
  Movement: Start the lift by un-racking the weight and holding it above your head or chest at a full extension. (2) Lower the bar down until it contacts your upper chest, keeping the elbows pointing outward. (3) After contact with the chest, raise the bar back up to the starting position, extending your arms fully.
  Note: Because this is on an incline and involves more of your front deltoids, you will not be able to lift as much on this press as you would on the flat bench. This movement puts emphasis on the top portion of the chest so it should be done with a strict movement trying to make the bar touch the same part of the chest every repetition.

Parallel Bar Dips

Primary Purpose: Mid-Chest
Secondary Purpose: Triceps

Function: On a dip bar, hold yourself up with your arms extended and cross your feet behind you.

Movement: Lower your body down as far as you can; lean slightly forward. (2) Press your body back to the starting position.

Note: To increase the intensity, you may use a dip belt and add weight to it. (2) You may also hold a dumbbell in between the legs or feet. (3) The further forward you lean; the more chests you incorporate.

Barbell Decline Bench Press

Primary Purpose: Lower Chest
Secondary Purpose: Triceps
Function: Lie on a decline bench approximately 30-40 degrees and grip the bar outside of shoulder width, with an overhand neutral grip and feet between the holders to prevent sliding.

Movement: Start the lift by un-racking the weight and holding it above your lower chest at a full extension. (2) Lower the bar down until it contacts your sternum area, keeping the elbows pointing outward. (3) After contact with the chest, raise the bar back up to the starting position, extending your arms fully.

Note: Because of the angle of this exercise, the range of motion is limited. Take advantage by bringing the bar as close to under your chest as possible, without irritating the shoulder.

Push-ups

Primary Purpose: Mid-Chest
Secondary Purpose: Triceps
Function: Lay on the floor face down with your hands on the side of you on the floor (shoulder width). Use your hands to push up to the top position, keeping your back straight.

Movement: Lower yourself down until your chest/torso slightly contacts the floor. (2) Push yourself back up to return to the top position, completing the rep.

Note: Some believe that you only need to go down until your arms break 90 degrees. However, I am a firm believer in getting a full range of motion during any exercise so that I am targeting every muscle fiber that is acclimated with that workout.

CHAPTER 12

LEGS

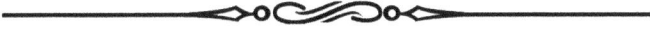

QUADRICEPS

HAMSTRING

CALF

GLUTEUS MAXIMUS

COMPOSITION OF THE LEGS

The separation of the legs refers to the quadriceps (front area of the thigh), hamstrings (rear area of the thigh), and the calve muscle. The legs being one of the biggest muscle groups of the body are targeted through different positioning of the feet. The quadriceps have four heads which are the rectus femoris, vastus intermedius (which makes the central part of the thigh), the vastus medialis (inner part of the thigh), and the vastus lateralis (outer part of the thigh).

The hamstring is known as the leg biceps as it is activated by curling movements for the legs. The hamstring muscle development consists of the bicep femoris, semitendinosus, and the semimembranosus. This muscle is right below the buttocks (gluteus maximus). Lastly, is the calve muscle which consists of the soleus (the large part of the calf) starting at the fibula and tibia and the gastrocnemius. The tibialis anterior runs from the front of the lower leg along the shin bone.

ACTIVATION OF THE MUSCLE

This muscle is generally activated by pushing movements with the legs.

Quadricep Exercises- Squats, Leg Press, Goblet Squats, Dumbbell Lunges, Front Squats, Leg Extension.

Hamstring Exercises- Straight Leg Dead-Lifts, Leg Curls

Calf Exercises- Calf raises with Dumbbells, Smith Machine, Calf Machine, or a Barbell.

LEG EXERCISES

Barbell Squat

Primary Purpose: All 4 heads of the Quadriceps

Secondary Purpose: Gluteal Muscles and Hamstrings

Function: Position yourself under a barbell resting on a squat rack with the barbell resting behind your head on your trapezius muscle. (2) Place your hands on the bar and ensure your legs are shoulder width apart with your feet facing slightly outside. (3) Keeping your head and chest up, un-rack the weight and take 1-2 steps back.

Movement: Bend your knees, keeping your torso upright until your thighs are parallel to the floor or lower. (2) Reverse the movement by pushing through your heels to return to the starting position.

Note: Wider stance works the inside of your thigh more. (2) Narrow stance works the outside of your thigh more. (3) Heavier weight may require you to use a belt.

Barbell Front Squat

Primary Purpose: Emphasis on Quadriceps

Secondary Purpose: Gluteal Muscles and Hamstrings

Function: Position yourself under a barbell, resting on a squat rack with the barbell resting on your upper pectorals and front deltoids. (2) Hold the bar with an overhand grip with your feet shoulder-width apart.

(3) Raise your chest and elbows as high as possible to ensure the barbell does not slide forward as you are un-racking the weight. (4) Un-rack the weight and take 1-2 steps back.

Movement: Bend your knees, keeping your torso upright until your thighs are parallel to the floor or lower. (2) Reverse the movement by pushing through your heels to return to the starting position.

Notes: Slightly arch your lower back as you are un-racking the weight. (2) Because the barbell is resting on the front side of the body as opposed to the back, you will naturally do less weight on this exercise than you can do on traditional squats.

Dumbbell Squat

Primary Purpose- Quadriceps
Secondary Purpose- Gluteal Muscles and Hamstrings
Function- Hold a dumbbell in each hand at your side with a neutral grip.

Movement- With your head and chest up, bend your knees keeping your torso upright until your thighs are parallel to the floor or lower. (2) Reverse the movement by pushing through your heels to return to the starting position.

Leg press

NOTE- The primary purpose depends on the position of the feet. Quadriceps will always be affected. However, other variations can promote stress on the other muscle as well.

Primary Purpose- Quadriceps
Secondary Purpose- Gluteal Muscles and Hamstrings
Function- Position yourself on a leg press machine with your back against the backrest and feet slightly apart on the footplate. (2) Pushing the weight up and holding the weight with your legs, unlock the safety hooks.

Movement- Bend your knees, lowering the weight until your thighs are touching your torso. (2) Press the weight back up through your heels until your legs are extended without locking your knees.

Note: Try to prevent yourself from putting your hands on your knees to assist with the lift. (2) The higher your feet on the foot plate, the more the gluteal muscles and hamstrings are being used. (3) The lower your feet on the footplate, the more the quadriceps are being used. (4) The further apart your feet on the footplate, the more the inside of your quadriceps are being used.

Lunge with the Barbell

Primary Purpose- Quadriceps
Secondary Purpose- Glutes
Function- Holding a barbell across the trapezius muscle behind your head, stand with your feet together.
Movement- Step forward with one foot leading with your heel, while lowering the other knee until it touches the floor. At this point, the front leg should be at 90 degrees. (2) Push yourself back up using the front heel, returning to the standing position, and bring your back leg to meet the front one. (3) Step forward with the other foot and repeat the movement, alternating legs.
Note: All repetitions can be done with one leg first then with the other or alternating. (2) This movement can be done using dumbbells as well.

Leg Extension

Primary Purpose- To define the Quadriceps
Secondary Purpose- N/A
Function- Sit with your back resting on the seat of the leg extension machine and your feet secured with the foot pads.
Movement- Extend your legs until the point of full extension, contracting your quads. (2) Slowly lower weight back down until your feet align with your knees.
Note: This exercise is designed for the definition of the quadriceps. Instead of worrying about how heavy you are lifting on this exercise, focus on the contraction you are getting with the movement.

Leg Curls

Primary Purpose- Hamstrings
Secondary Purpose- N/A
Function- Lay on a leg curl machine with your legs under the foot padding.
Movement- Pushing your chest up off the pad slightly, curl your legs up as far as possible to the point where your heel is almost in contact with your buttocks/lower back. (2) Lower the weight back down controllably emphasizing on the eccentric movement of the exercise.
Note: N/A

Straight Leg Dead-Lifts

Primary Purpose- Hamstrings
Secondary Purpose- Gluteus Maximus and lower back
Function- With your feet roughly shoulder width apart, grab a barbell with a mixed grip or overhand grip and stand with the bar in front of your thighs as if you just completed a deadlift.
Movement- Keeping your legs straight (without locking your knees), bend forward at the hips, and lower your torso until parallel with the floor, keeping the bar at arm's length. (2) Reverse the movement to return back to the starting position.
Note: Ensure your back is kept straight and not rounded during this movement. (2) The bar should always be positioned over the toe when lowering the weight. (3) This exercise can be done standing on top of a bench or box for maximum effectiveness.

CHAPTER 13

ARMS

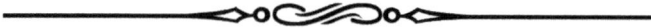

BICEPS

TRICEPS

FOREARMS

COMPOSITION OF THE ARMS

The separation of arms consists of three major muscle groups. The biceps, the triceps, and the forearm. The bicep is a muscle with two heads (biceps branchii long head and short head), which begins underneath the front deltoid. It provides a function for curl movements to be activated. Next, is the triceps. This is a three-headed muscle that is opposed to the bicep. The triceps consist of the lateral head, the long head, and the medial head. Lastly is the forearm. This is the lower part of the arm consisting of flexors and extensors.

ACTIVATION OF THE MUSCLE

The bicep muscle is generally activated by "pulling" movements

NOTE: To work the inner area of your biceps (short head), use a wider grip with your movement. (2) To work the outer area of your biceps (long head), use a closer grip with your movement.

The triceps muscle is generally activated by "pushing" movements

NOTE: With the triceps being 2/3 of your arms circumference, I recommend training your triceps more vigorously than your biceps due to the fact that it will require more attention because of its size in relation to the bicep.

Bicep Exercises- Dumbbell curls, Barbell curls, Incline curls, Hammer curls.

Triceps Exercises- Dumbbell kickbacks, Triceps Extensions, Dips, Skull-Crushers

Forearm Exercises- Hammer Curls, Dumbbell Wrist Curls, Reverse Curls

BICEPS EXERCISES

DUMBBELL CURL (STANDING OR SEATED)

Primary Purpose: Biceps
Secondary Purpose: Slightly Front Delt
Function: Stand or sit with a dumbbell in each hand. (2) With your feet shoulder-width apart, bend slightly forward at the hips.

Movement: Without rocking, curl the dumbbell (twisting it as far as possible), as you are raising it towards your front deltoids. (2) Lower the dumbbell back to your sides keeping tension on your biceps on the way down.

Note: As you curl the weight towards your shoulders, your palms should face you. (2) As you reach the top of the movement, ensure you twist the dumbbell, bringing your pinky as far towards you as possible to capitalize on the contraction. (3) This exercise can be done in different variations. You can alternate one hand at a time, both hands and curl simultaneously or you can do one arm until the completed amount of reps then do the other.

BARBELL CURL

Primary Purpose: Biceps

Function: Using an underhand grip, hold a barbell in front of your thighs with your hands shoulder-width apart.

Movement: Without rocking, curl the barbell towards your front deltoids. (2) Lower the barbell back to your thighs controllably keeping tension on your biceps on the way down.

Note: Try to keep your elbows fixed at your sides. (2) This exercise has strict movement on the wrist so you may also use an e-z bar for this exercise.

INCLINE DUMBBELL CURL

Primary Purpose: Biceps

Function: Laying on an incline bench at roughly a 45-degree angle, hold a dumbbell in each hand at your side with a neutral grip.

Movement: Keeping your palms face up and your shoulder blades pinched together, curl both of the dumbbells towards your front delt without lifting your elbows. (2) Lower the weight back down to your side, returning to the starting position.

Note: Try to keep your elbows attached to your sides throughout the movement. For a deeper contraction, pull the elbows back so that you can bring the dumbbells right below the armpit area. (2) Fully extend the rep at the bottom to stretch the bicep to its full capacity.

PREACHER CURL

Primary Purpose: Biceps

Function: Sit on a preacher curl bench with an E-Z bar resting on the rack. (2) Placing your elbows on the pad, grab the E-Z bar with an underhand grip (the inside grip works the outside of your bicep while the outside grip works the inside of your bicep).

Movement: Curl the E-Z bar to your shoulders. (2) Lower the weight back down controllably to a full extension and then repeat.

Note: To increase the intensity of this exercise, put your feet behind you and let the pad rest under your armpit area prior to lifting the E-Z bar and completing reps.

DUMBBELL HAMMER CURL

Primary Purpose: Long head of biceps
Secondary Purpose: Forearms
Function: Hold dumbbells at your side with a neutral grip (palms face the body).
Movement: Lift the dumbbells up towards your front deltoids while keeping your hands in the same position they started in throughout the movement. (2) Lower the weight back down slowly until arms are fully extended.
Note: This movement can be done seated or standing. (2) This exercise can also be done where you cross the dumbbells to the opposite shoulder (across the body).

CONCENTRATION CURL

Primary Purpose: Peak of the bicep
Function: Sitting on a bench, hold a dumbbell in one hand with that elbow resting on the inside of the thigh on the same side. (2) Put your free arm on the unoccupied leg for support.
Movement: Bending slightly forward, curl the dumbbell up to your shoulders while keeping the elbow positioned on the thigh. As you are lifting, twist the wrist so that your pinky is the highest finger at the top of the rep. (2) Lower the weight back down to the full extension.
Note: Ensure you are bringing the weight to your shoulder and not to your chest.

TRICEP EXERCISES

CABLE PUSHDOWNS

Primary Purpose: Triceps
Function: Connect the attachment of choice to a pulley machine (straight bar or v-bar). (2) Grab the bar with an overhand grip.

Movement: With your elbows tucked at your side and knees slightly bent, press the weight down to a full extension. Your chest should remain up to ensure you are not using your body weight to assist you with the lift. (2) With your arms fully extended, come back up only until your arm makes a 90-degree angle. This will allow you to keep tension on the triceps throughout the movement. (3) Repeat the next rep, only returning to the 90-degree angle until the set is completed.

Note: By coming up more than 90 degrees, you relieve your triceps of some tension and may add a bit of shoulder to assist you with the lift. Also, at 90 degrees, the momentum that you will normally get from the extended rep will be cut in half, allowing you to generate more power in a shorter movement. (2) The full range of motion will work the lower triceps more efficiently if that is your focus. (3) This exercise can be done with multiple attachments. Typically, I would recommend a short bar or the v-bar but you may also use a LAT-pulldown bar or the rope, which will focus more on the lateral head of the triceps.

SINGLE-ARM REVERSE PUSHDOWN

Primary Purpose: Lateral head of the triceps
Secondary Purpose: Medial and long head of the triceps.
Function: Grab a D-grip attachment on an overhead pulley with a reverse grip (palms facing up). (2) Keep your chest up and bend slightly at the knees.
Movement: With your elbows tucked to the side, press the weight down to a full extension. (2) With your arms fully extended, come back up only until your arms make a 90-degree angle. This will allow you to keep tension on the triceps throughout the movement. (3) Repeat the next rep, only returning to the 90-degree angle until the set is completed.
Note: Try to keep your elbows fixed at your sides and hold the contraction for about 1-2 seconds at the bottom of every rep.

DUMBBELL KICKBACKS

Primary Purpose: Upper area of triceps

Function: Stand with your knees slightly bent with one foot in front of the other. (2) Leaning forward at the waist, have a dumbbell in the hand on the same side foot that it is in the rear. (3) Place the other hand on your opposite knee or on a bench.

Movement: Lift your elbow up and keep it tucked near your torso and the extend the dumbbell fully. At the end of the extension, your palms should be face up. (2) Complete the designated number of reps with one arm and then continue to the other arm.

Note: Try to keep your elbows attached to your side throughout the movement.

LYING TRICEPS EXTENSIONS (SKULLCRUSHERS)

Primary Purpose: Long head of triceps

Function: Using an E-Z bar, lay flat on a bench with your head hanging slightly off the end and your feet planted on the ground. (2) With an overhand grip, hold the weight above your head but behind the head at roughly a 45-degree angle.

Movement: Keeping your elbows in place, lower the weight down to your head and then press back up to the starting position.

Note: Be careful not to let the weight hit you in the forehead. Control the weight throughout the repetition. (2) Lowering the weight at an angle behind your head works the long head of the triceps. Bringing the bar to your forehead keeps tension on the medial and lateral heads of the triceps.

LYING DUMBELL TRICEP EXTENSIONS

Primary Purpose: Triceps

Function: Lie flat on a bench holding dumbbells in each hand with a neutral grip and your feet planted on the floor.

Movement: With your arms held straight and palms facing one another, lower the weight by bending at the elbow until both dumbbells are beside your head. (2) Press the weight back up to a full lockout, keeping the dumbbells at an angle behind the head.

DIPS

Primary Purpose: Triceps
Function: Hold yourself up on the parallel bars
Movement: Lower yourself down as far as you can go, keeping your torso and your legs aligned straight up. (2) From the lower position, press your body back up until you are back at the starting position.
Note: This exercise can be done with a weight belt to increase the intensity. (2) Leaning back adds emphasis on the triceps. Leaning forward adds emphasis on the chest.

CLOSE GRIP BENCH PRESS

Primary Purpose: Triceps
Secondary Purpose: Front Delts
Function: Lie on a bench and grip the bar inside of shoulder width, with an overhand neutral grip and feet planted on the floor.
Movement: Start the lift by un-racking the weight and holding it above your head at a full extension. (2) Lower the bar down until it contacts right below your sternum, keeping the elbows tucked by your side. (3) After contact with the chest, raise the bar back up to the starting position, extending your arms fully.
Note: This exercise can be used strategically as it is one of the heaviest lifts the triceps can endure.

CHAPTER 14

BIG 3

———◦◦◦———

(BENCH PRESS, DEADLIFT, AND SQUAT)

BENCH PRESS

THE BENCH PRESS. Known as the upper-body monster; who wouldn't want to have an impressive bench? This is a lift used by almost all athletes to build strength and power. Out of your three main lifts, this will probably be the one you stagnate at first. I will say that nine times out of ten, this is because the supporting muscles such as the triceps, forearms, and shoulders are underdeveloped and not as big as the muscles which support squats and deadlifts such as the legs and the back.

Properly developing these supporting muscles can be the primary factor in increasing your bench press. Having a huge bench press is something that is impressive in the gym environment but I would like you to consider the riskiness of the actual lift to ensure that form is never compromised. To put it in context, the lift consists of hoisting hundreds of pounds over your neck and chest area where on little slip can result in a critical injury. Though a favorable exercise, its complexity is often overlooked.

WARM-UP: Prior to getting under the bar, prepare to lift it to glorify your strength, take 2-5 minutes at least to warm up your shoulders. During warm-ups, you do not want to incorporate too much triceps because it may cause fatigue so my recommendation would be to reframe from pressing movements. In this case, dumbbell lateral and front raises are just fine.

My experience has been that when my rotator cuff and shoulders feel healthy, my bench press days are significantly better. Taking the warm-up a step further, you can get on a bench and push an empty bar, simulating a bench press and controlling the path of the bar to determine your comfort levels. You practice the way you perform so you do not throw the bar up and down just because no weight is on it. Take your time in actually trying to contract the muscle of focus; the chest.

GRIP: Many people believe that the more triceps they incorporate, the heavier they will be able to lift. Let's not forget that this exercise is designed for your chest. That being said, shoulder width is ideal. In some cases, I will actually recommend going slightly outside of shoulder width just to activate the outer pectorals a little more. The closer your hands are placed, the more the triceps are involved.

As you grab the bar, assure your thumb is wrapped around the bar so that you can squeeze the bar. Executing this lift using the "false grip" where your thumb does not wrap around is way too unsafe for you to be worrying about putting any weight on the bar. Like I said before, one slip can be a very damaging mistake.

I find that the tighter grip I have on the bar the more power I can generate. Reframe from excessive bending at the wrist. Your wrist cannot hold as much weight as your forearms can, being it is a joint. Keeping your wrist locked will allow the weight to be distributed to your forearms and then to the triceps. If you have a habit of popping or turning your wrist during your lift, I will recommend that you use wrist straps to help reiterate the importance of supporting your wrists.

FORM AND LIFT: As you lay on a bench, position yourself so that your eyes are roughly in line with the bar. Place your hands on the bar about shoulder-width apart. Once in position, pinch your shoulder blades together which will help you flare out your LATS, keeping your shoulder blades pressed against the bench.

Naturally, this should create a natural arch in the small of your back. Keep your feet planted flat on the ground. This will allow you to generate extra power and is used as a form of stability. Take the bar off of the rack and center it roughly above your lower chest. Descend down until the bar touches your chest. Push the bar back up to the starting position. Re-rack the weight.

REST: Before completing your next set, you need roughly a 2-3 minute break to let your muscle fibers recoup.

DEADLIFTS

THE DEADLIFT. When you walk into a gym and load up a barbell with plates on top of plates, you cannot help but be noticed. A deadlift by far is one of the most impressive lifts to watch. Being that it is a full-body exercise, this workout exerts mass bodybuilding. This lift is how you test your ultimate strength.

WARM-UP: Prior to hoisting some heavy weight off of the floor, be sure to warm up your lower back. You can do this by holding dumbbells in your hands and trying to "touch your toes" with them or some simple good mornings. You may also use an empty barbell and simulate doing a deadlift. There is no better way to warm up than by performing the actual lift in simulation with no weight.

As you begin putting weight on the bar, concentrate on keeping your form strict while the weight is still light. People have bad tendencies of lifting the light weight just to get to the bigger weight, failing to activate the actual muscles required to lift the heavy weight. The same way you do the light weight is the same way you should do the heavy weight.

GRIP: When grabbing the bar, the best grip to use is a mixed grip. This is done by grabbing the bar with one hand in an overhand position and the opposing hand holding the bar with an underhand grip. There are multiple variations to deadlifts that may require you to hold the bar differently but the most ideal is a mixed grip to prevent the bar from slipping when being lifted.

FORM AND LIFT: As you stand with the bar in front of you, the standard lift would require that your legs are shoulder width apart unless you are doing sumo deadlifts or Romanian deadlifts. My experience has taught me that when people have their feet widely apart, as the weight gets heavier, they start incorporating their lower back. Lower back soreness is very irritating and actually shies people away from doing deadlifts in the first place. To prevent this, I recommend bringing your feet closer together. This will allow you to put your buttocks down more as if you are getting ready to sit in a chair.

If done correctly, the bottom portion of the lift should require you to use a majority of your legs to break the weight off the ground. At the point the bar reaches your knee, you should be pulling your shoulder blades back. The bar may slide slightly up your thigh as if you are doing a row when you pull your shoulder blades back.

Think of how gravity works. Gravity pulls the weight downward (forward) so by pulling your shoulder blades back, tension will be on your back muscles. While pulling your shoulder blades back, you are standing up simultaneously. When you are close to the top of your rep, you will see that people have a tendency of thrusting their hips forward. This is incorrect.

At the top of your rep, the movement should feel as if you are trying to row the weight. This is actually you completing the shoulder blade pullback. Obviously, the heavier you go, the less dramatic this movement will look. However, the contraction will still be there.

To lower the weight, release your shoulder blades and lower the weight. When the bar reaches your knee, begin to squat down until the bar touches the floor. Do not lean over, letting the weight pull you. Instead, control the weight, bending at the knees as if you are trying to sit back in the chair again. Do not excessively bounce the weight off of the ground during your reps, as it will disengage your contraction for that slight second, which may cause an injury.

REST: Before completing your next set, you need roughly a 2-3 minute break to let your muscles recoup. As I mentioned before, form is compromised when exhaustion and fatigue is a factor. To prevent injury, use adequate rest periods.

INCREASE IN WEIGHT: As you increase in weight, be sure to measure the increments appropriately. Generally, on a deadlift, I will not recommend jumping in excess of 90 lbs at any given time. My highest deadlift to date is 605 lbs. I take full advantage of utilizing 25lb plates, 10lb plates, and even the 5lb plates after I pass 495 lbs. Though I can go from 495 lbs to 585 lbs in one set, I usually break it down into about 2 or maybe even 3 sets. 545lbs and then 565lbs and then 585lbs.

This allows me not only to get extra reps in but to also ensure that I am capable of holding form as I go up. Some days are better than others, so it is best to be safe every time by going up in smaller increments the closer you get to your 1RM. Once the weight gets heavy, all of the weight following is only going to be heavier, so it is imperative that form is never compromised. Not even for a new personal record.

SQUAT

THE SQUAT. Your legs are the foundation. Once your legs are strong, it will assist you in a majority of your other lifts. Being that your legs generates the most testosterone; one should take the squat very seriously to assist in growth. If you want to impress someone, try having some dominant legs. I know too many people with huge tops because all they do is chest, arms, and back, but when they wear shorts, it takes away from all they have worked hard for.

Everyone would shy away from chicken legs, but very few actually take the time to build their legs. This is where the squat comes in. The squat is one, if not the best leg building exercise. It focuses predominantly on the quads but also puts emphasis on the hamstrings and calves as well. It is mandatory that you do your squats correctly because a back injury is no joke. You have to consider the fact that squats consist of having hundreds of pounds resting on your spine. One slip or bad movement can end a workout career and leave you paralyzed.

WARM-UP: Prior to loading up a barbell with heavy weight, warm your legs up with just the bar or air squats. This will help warm up your knees and assure that you do not have any aches or pains. Again, there is no better way to warm up than by performing the actual lift in simulation with no weight.

GRIP: Place the bar so that it is resting on your trapezius muscle. Your hands should be placed shoulder width apart or wider with your feet aligned shoulder width apart as well.

FORM AND LIFT: As you stand up with the bar, un-racking it from the rack, take 2-3 steps back. Realign your feet so that they are shoulder width apart with your feet pointing very slightly towards the outside. Squat down from the hip as if you are trying to sit in a chair, keeping your chest and head raised up. If it helps, stare at one spot on the wall to ensure your head and chest are not lowering during the lift. As you reach 90 degrees or lower, push through your heels to return back up to a standing position. Re-rack the weight back on the squat rack.

INCREASE IN WEIGHT: Do not be afraid to use a belt to assist you in the lift. As you increase in weight, be sure to measure the increments appropriately. Generally, on a squat, the same rules apply in jumping weight as the deadlift. Your increase should not be in excess of 90 lbs at any given time. Utilize the smaller plates to your advantage. Too big of an increase can be a shock to your legs and lower back. Be safe every time by going up in smaller increments the closer that you get to your 1RM.

REST: Before completing your next set, you need roughly a 2-3 minute break to let your muscles recoup. As I mentioned before, form is compromised when exhaustion and fatigue are a factor. To prevent injury, allow adequate rest periods.

MAX CALCULATION SHEET

This sheet is a guideline to help you accurately perform your lifts based on percentages to get the most accurate and fastest results. With every exercise listed, you will calculate your 1RM (1 Rep Max) or 10RM (10 Rep Max) and use this sheet as your reference throughout the programs. To calculate a percent of your max, multiply your max by the number you are trying to figure out with a decimal in front of it.

Ex. Imagine your 1RM=315

If you were trying to find **55%** of **315lbs,** you should multiply 315 by .55 which will give you 173.25lbs. Calculate your percentages for the best results.

WORK-OUTS	50% 1 RM	55% 1 RM	60% 1 RM	65% 1 RM	70% 1 RM	75% 1 RM	80% 1 RM	85% 1 RM	90% 1 RM	95% 1 RM	1-1 RM
Flat Bench Press											
Incline Bench Press											

Decline Bench Press											
Squat											
Deadlift											
WORK-OUTS	50% 10 RM	55% 10 RM	60% 10 RM	65% 10 RM	70% 10 RM	75% 10 RM	80% 10 RM	85% 10 RM	90% 10 RM	95% 10 RM	1-10 RM
Flat Bench Dumb-ell Press (10 Rep Max)											
Incline Bench Dumb-ell Press (10 Rep Max)											
Decline Bench Dumb-ell Press (10 Rep Max)											
Leg Press (10 Rep Max)											

Dumb-bell Shoul-der Press (10 Rep Max)										

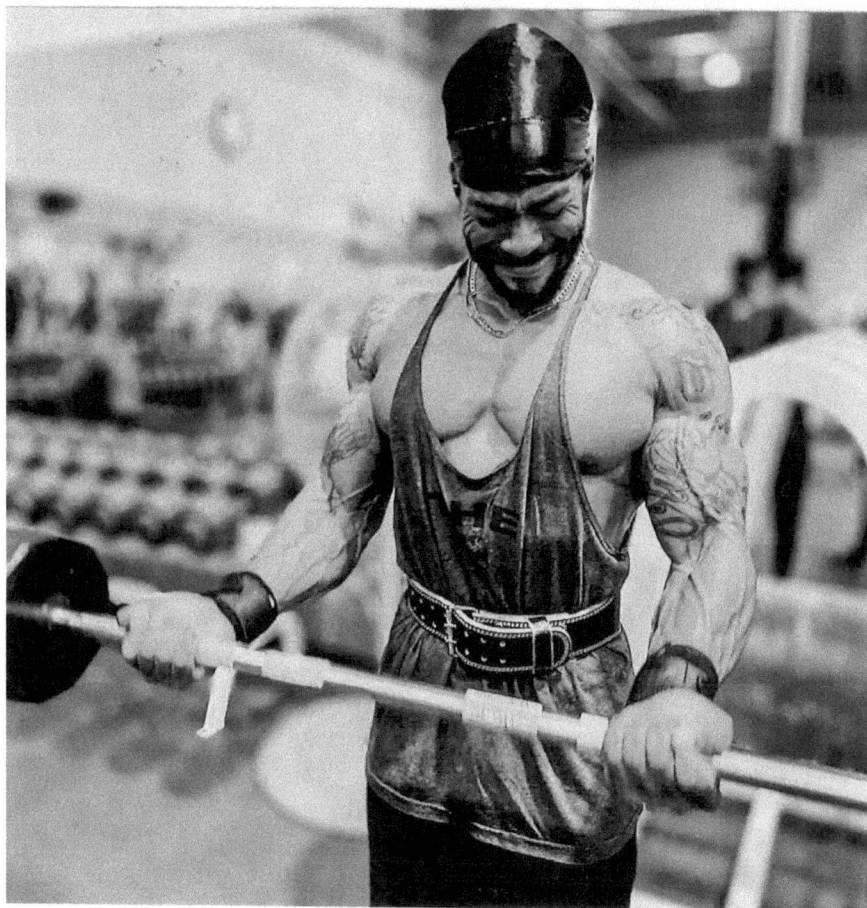

ARMS (Biceps) - Barbell Curl

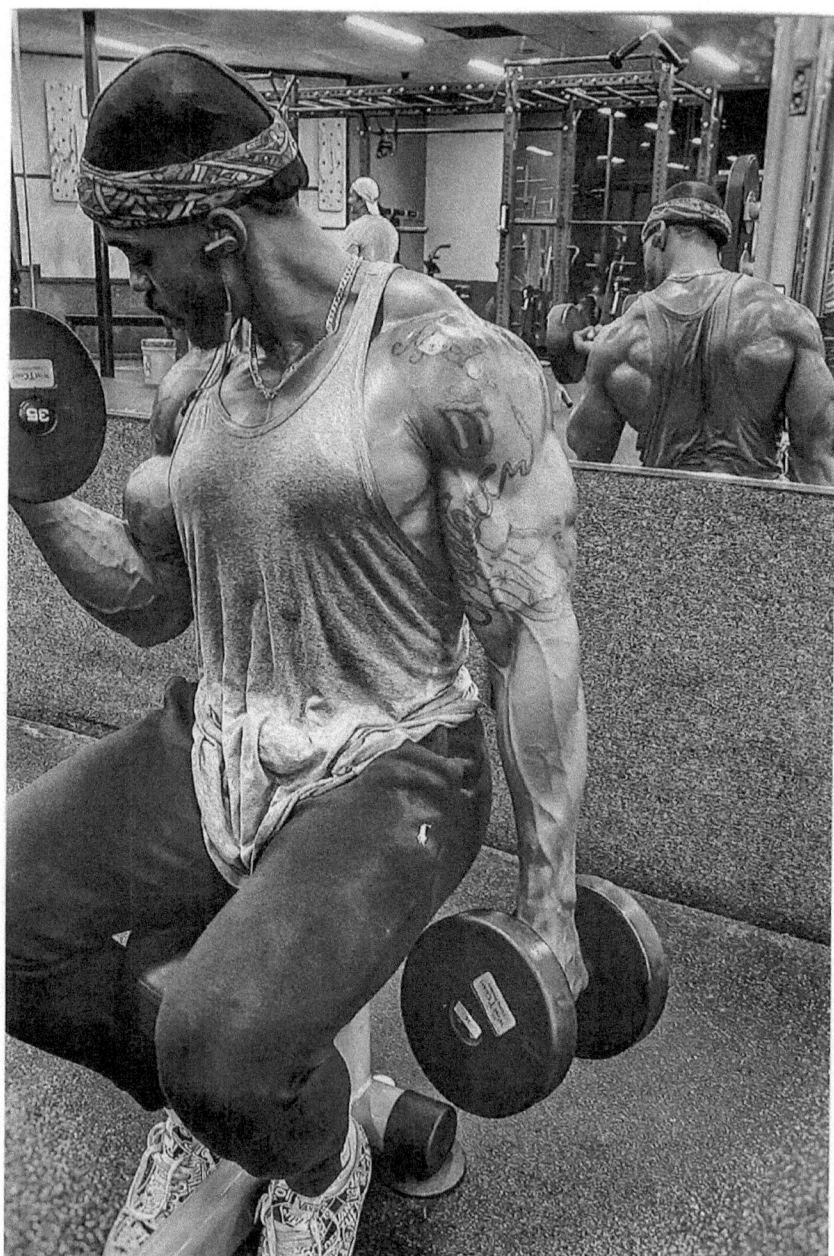

ARMS (Biceps) - Seated Dumbbell Curl

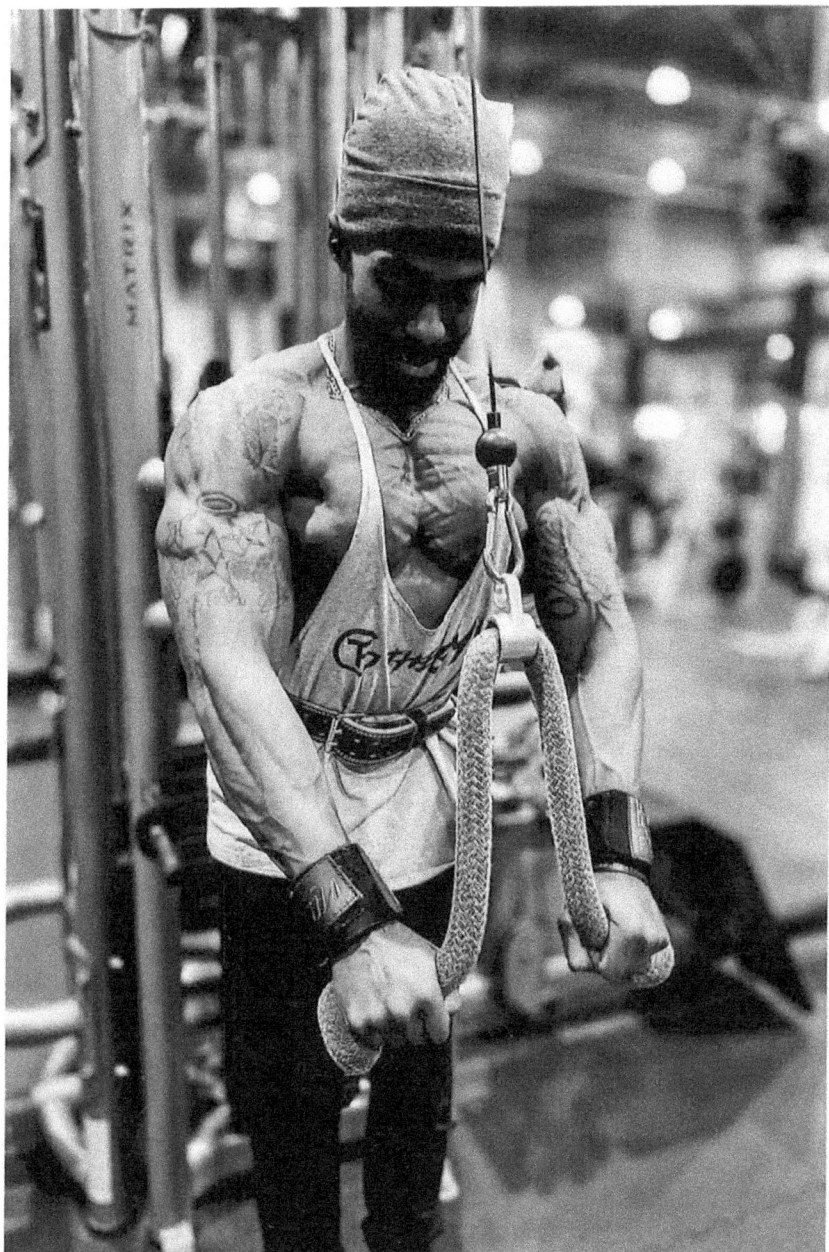

ARMS (Triceps) - Tricep Rope Extension (Bottom)

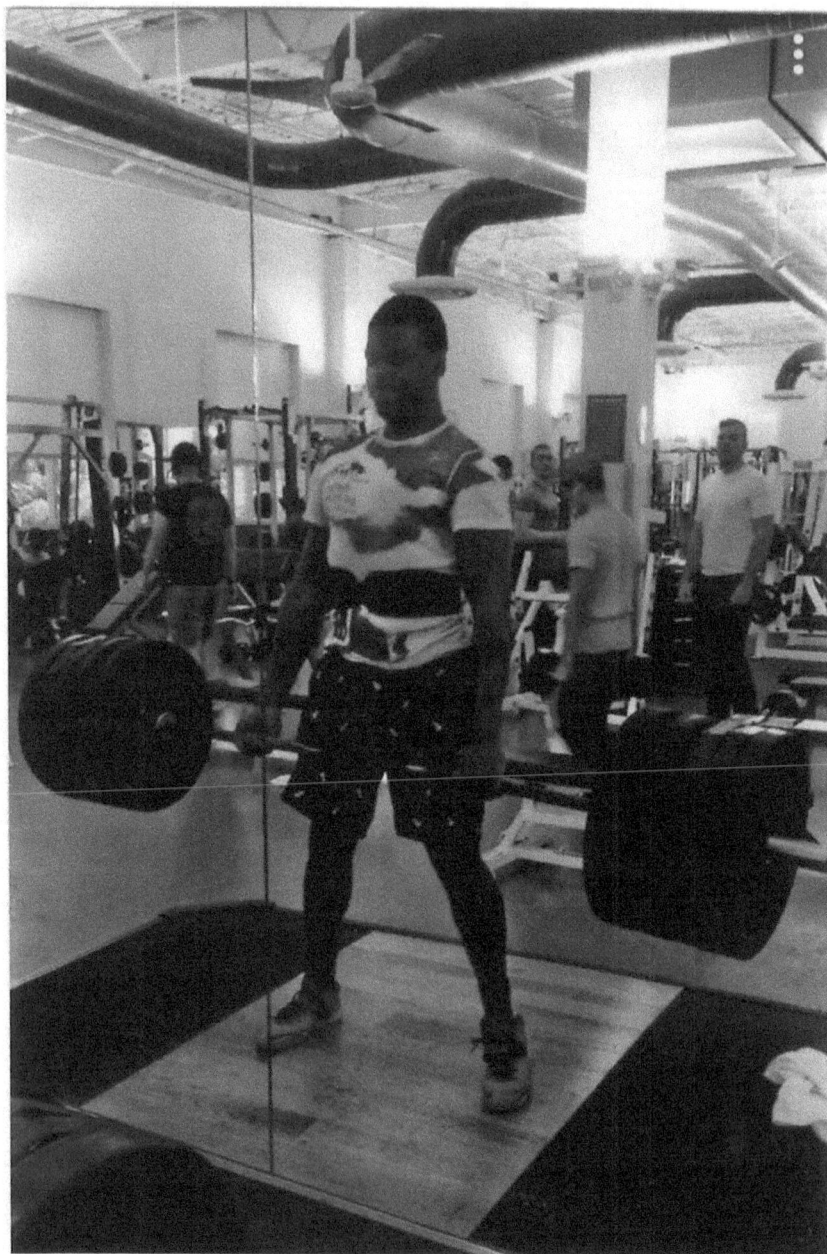

Author Deadlifting 495 lbs

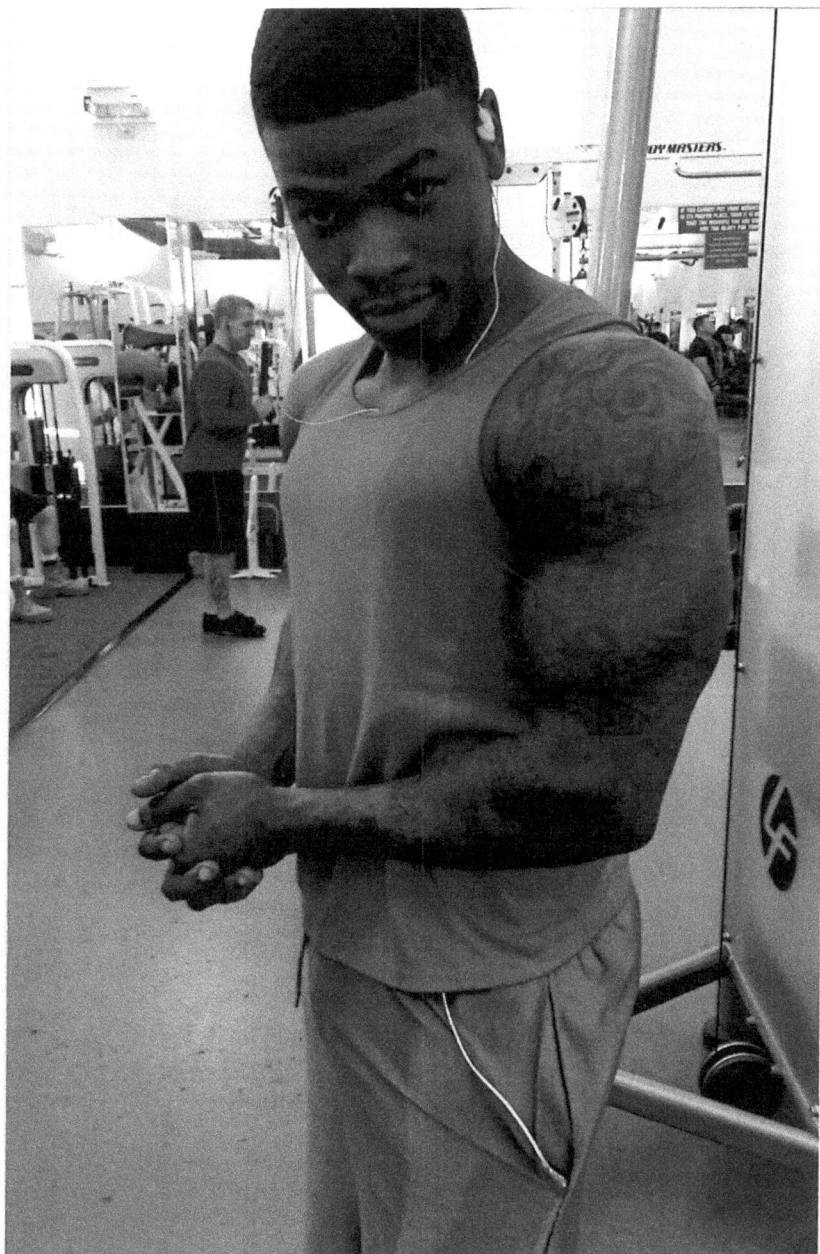

Author's physique before incarceration

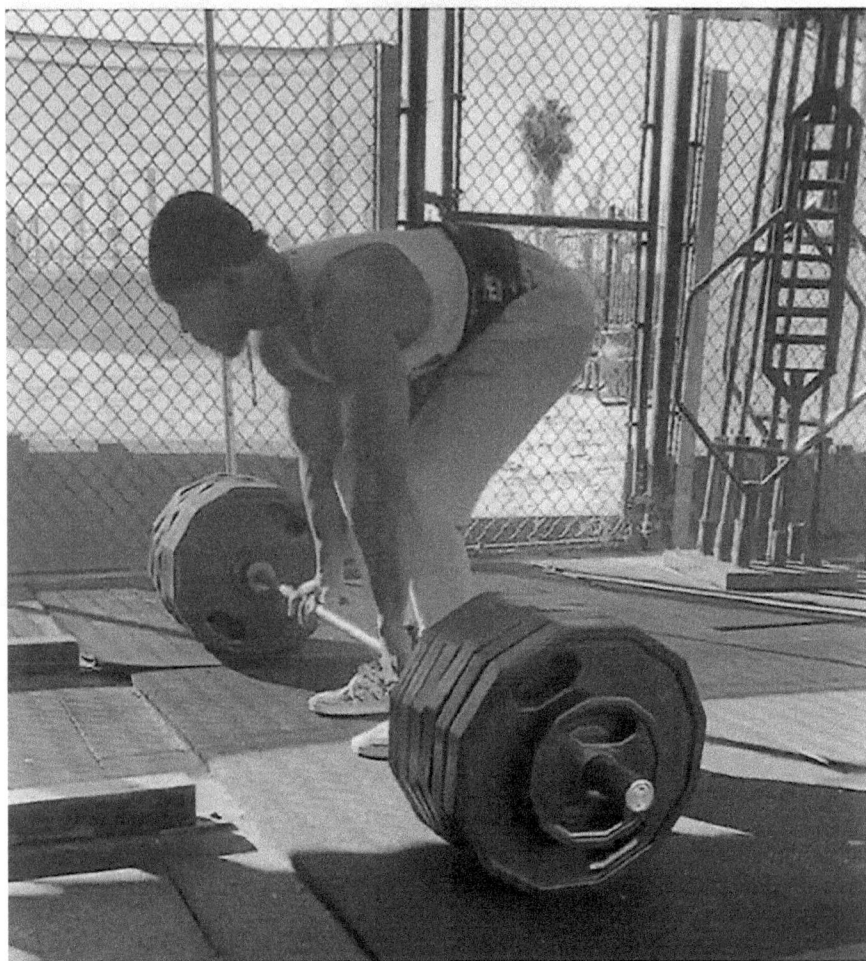

BACK - Deadlift #1 (bottom position)

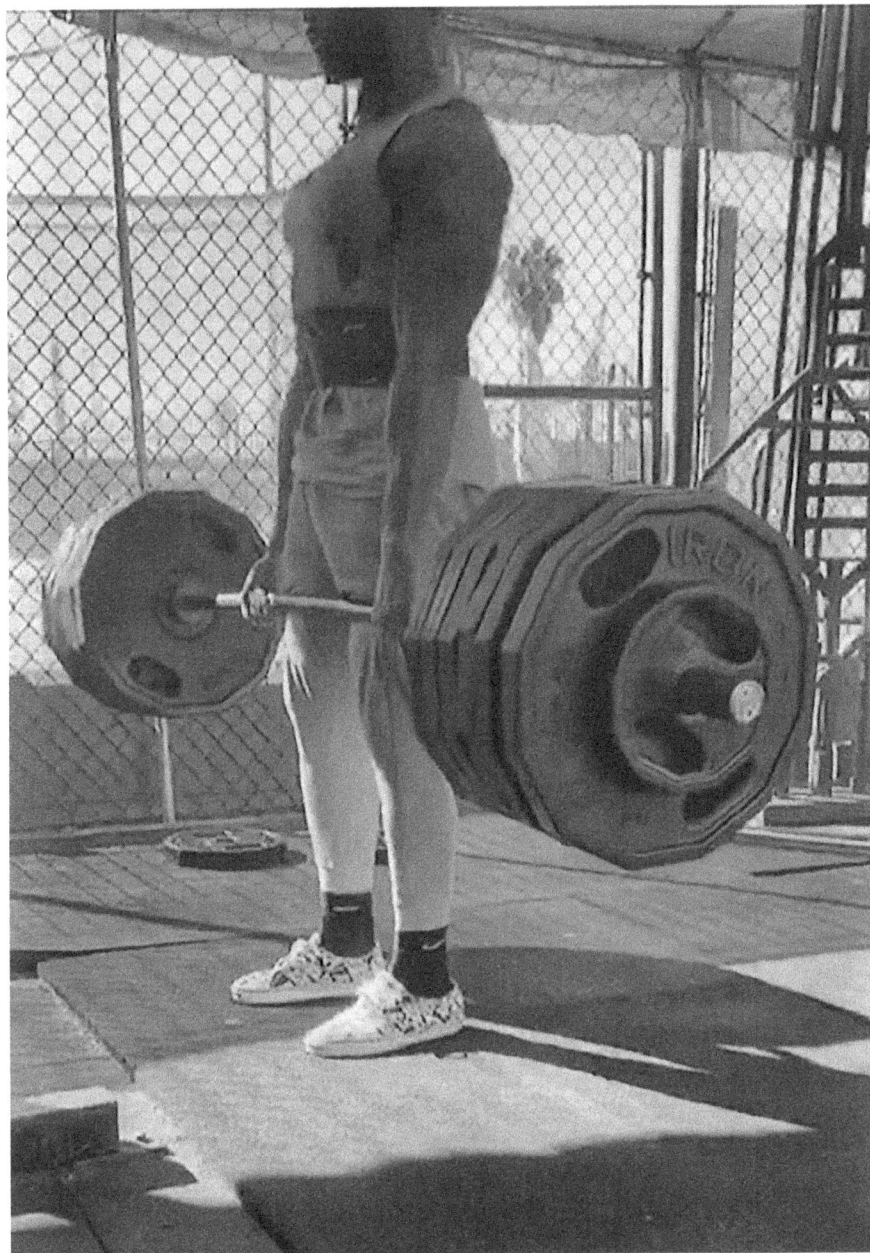

BACK - Deadlift #2 (top position)

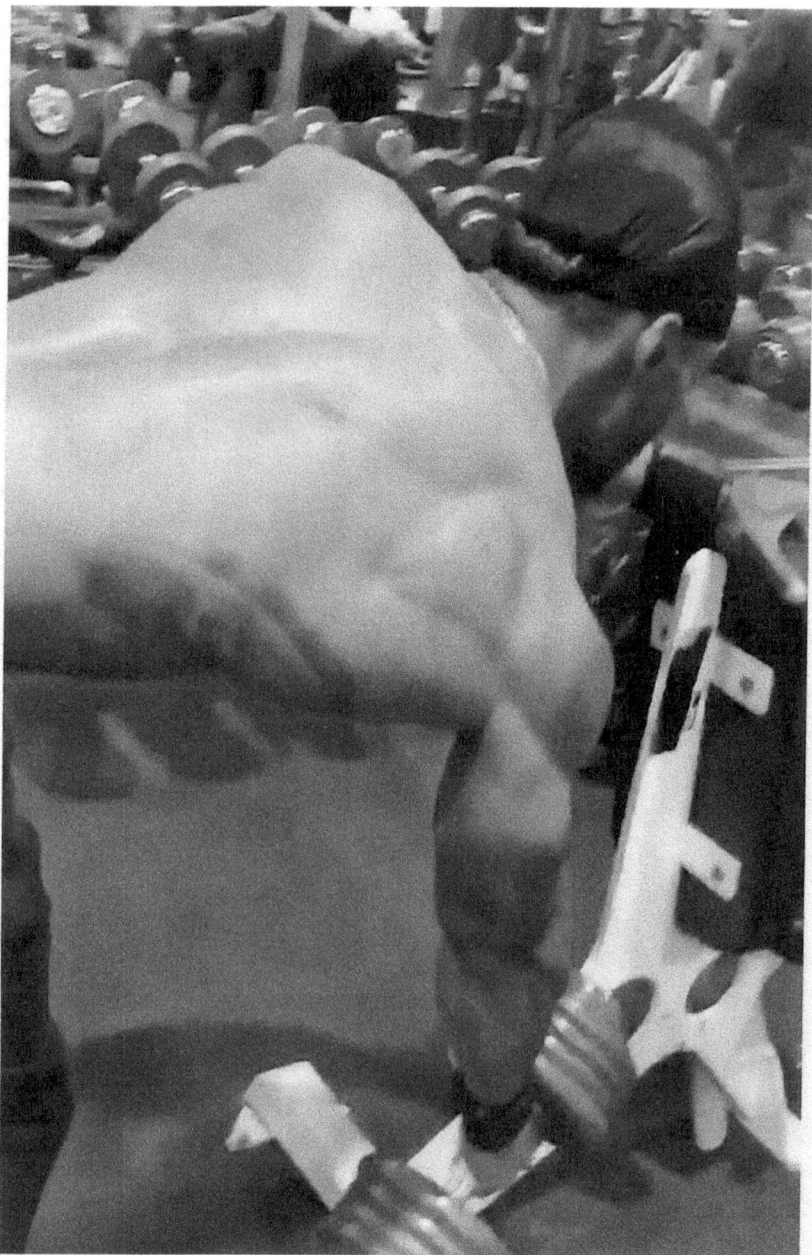

BACK - Dumbbell Row (bottom)

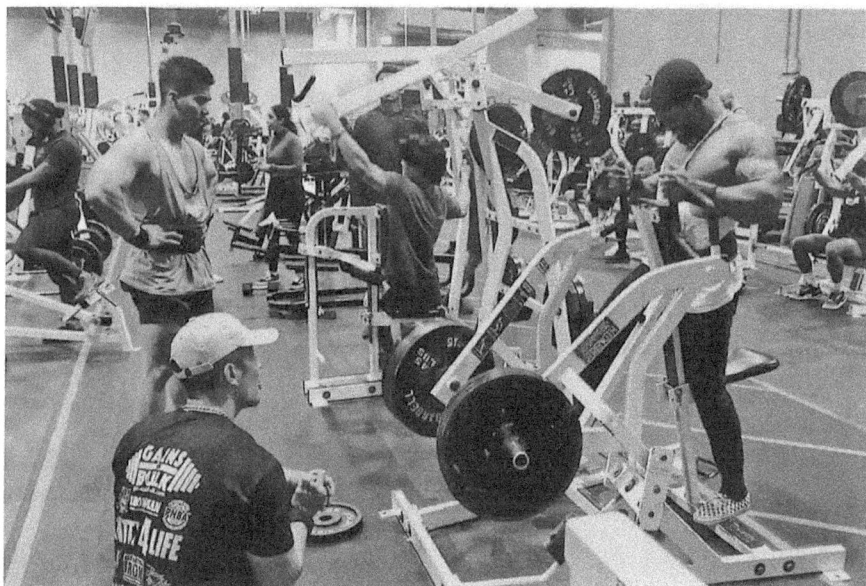

BACK - Row Machine

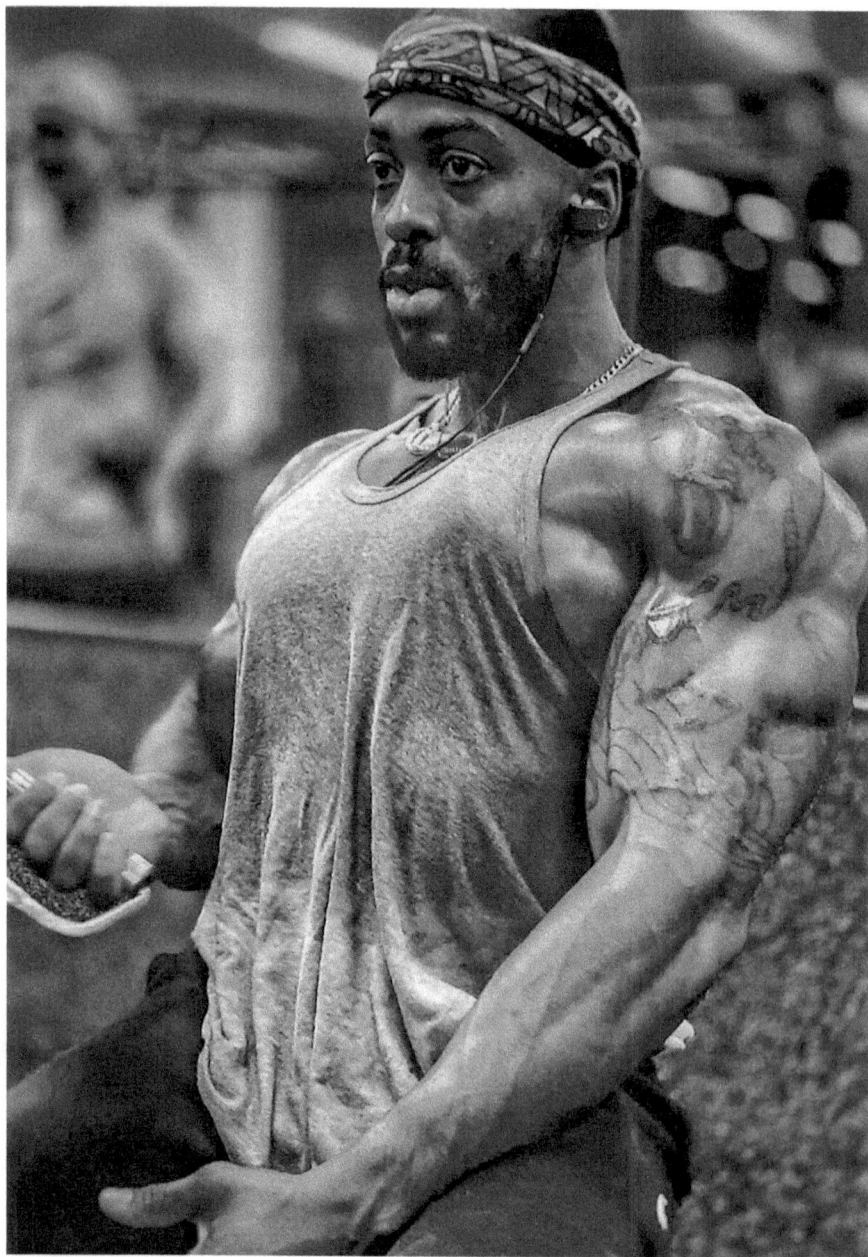

BACK - Single Arm Cable Row - Instagram - @djayretroflyy

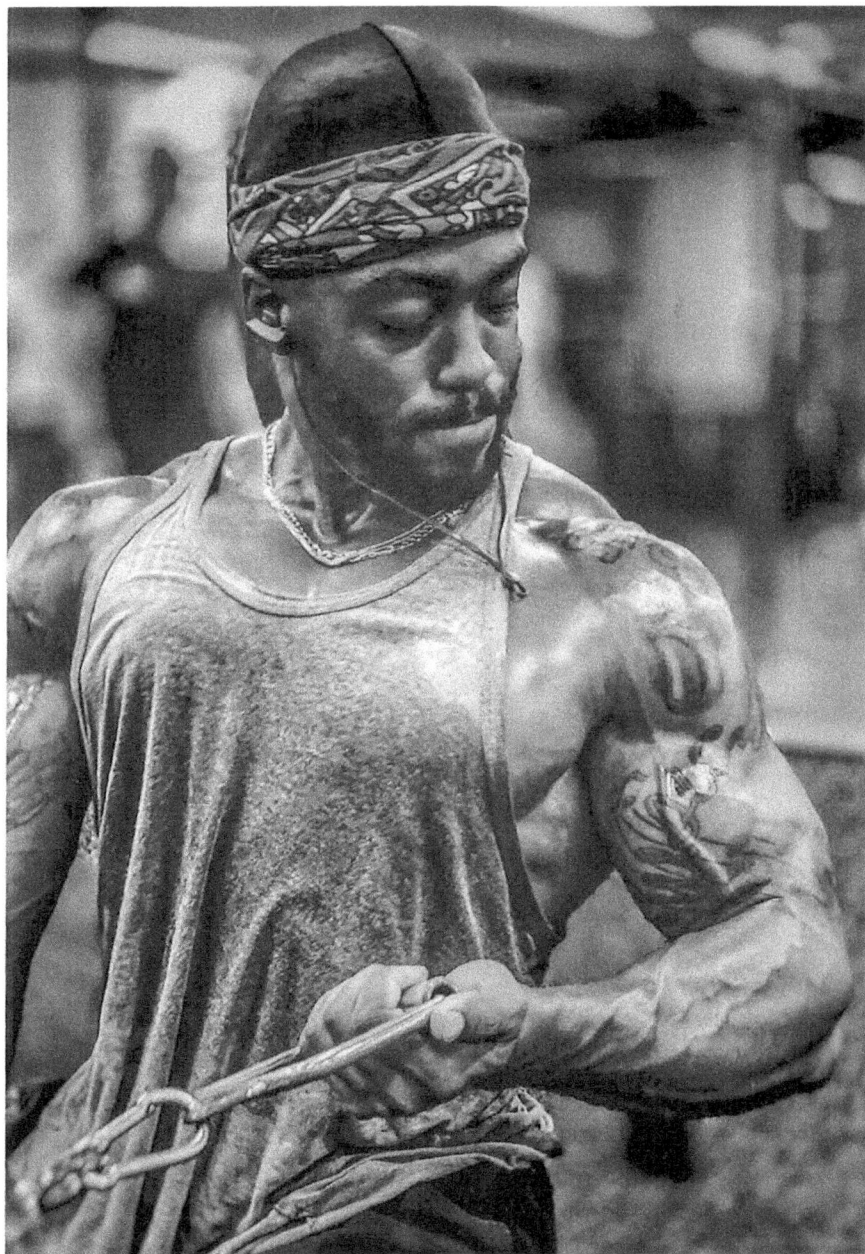

BACK - Single Arm Cable Row

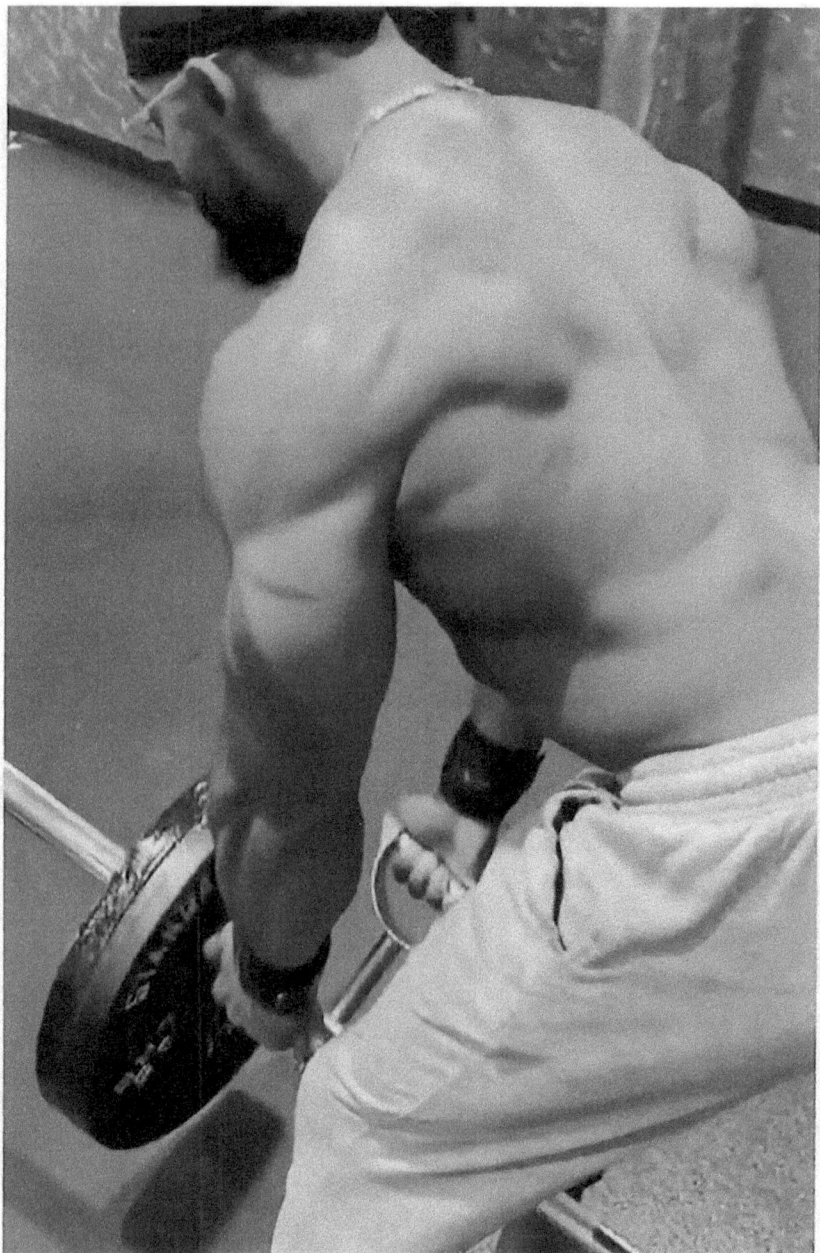

BACK - T-Bar Row (Bottom)

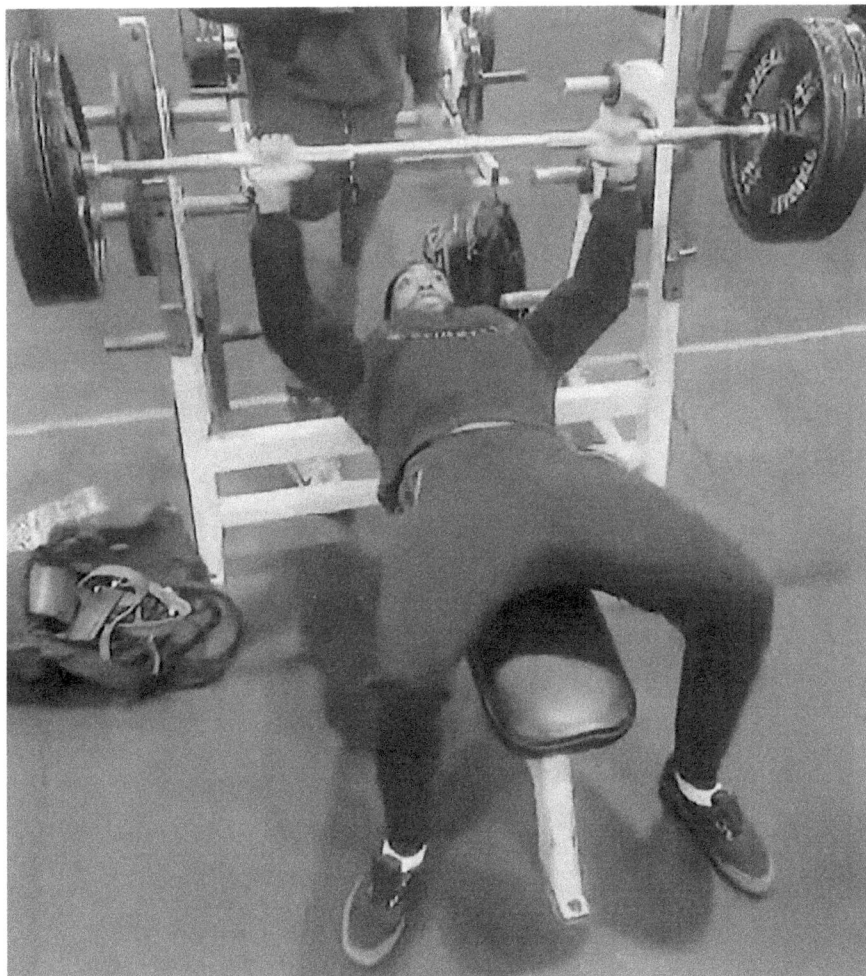

CHEST - Barbell Flat Bench Press (Top)

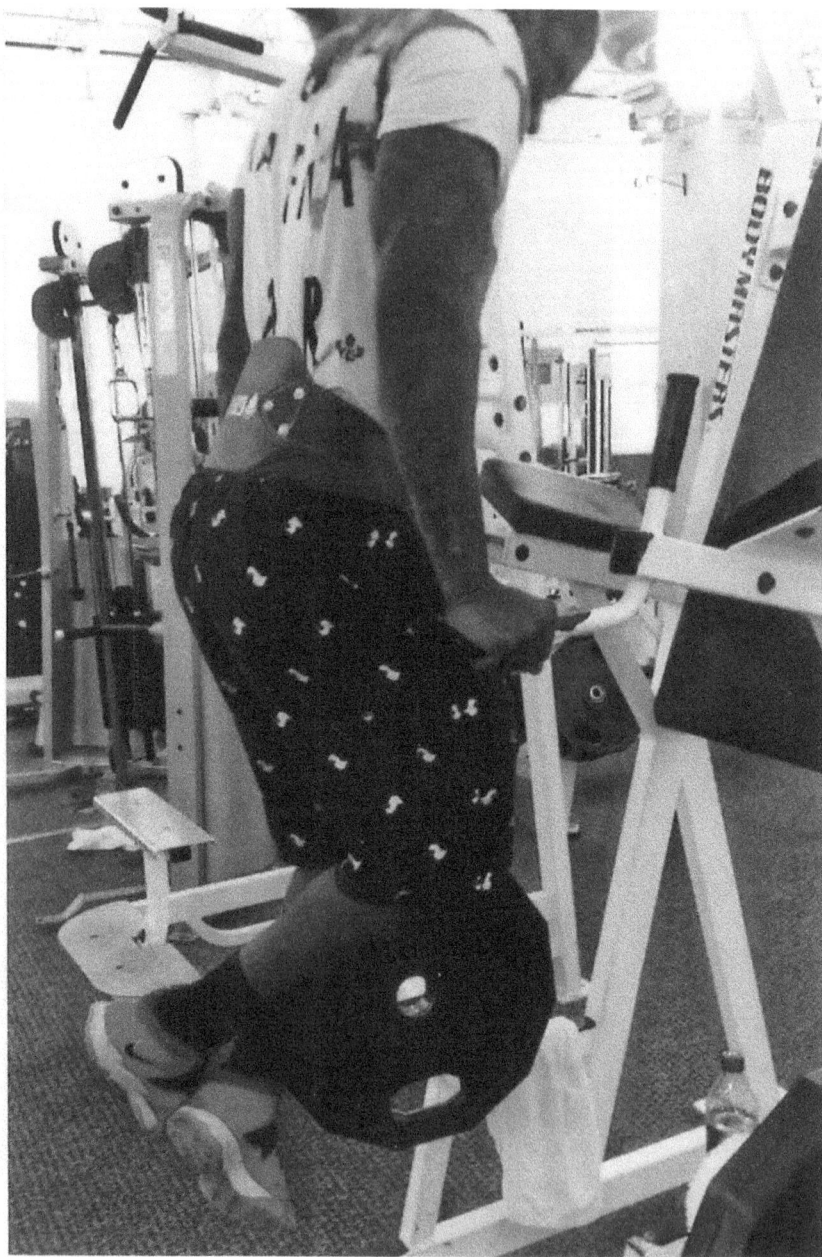

CHEST - *Weighted Dip*

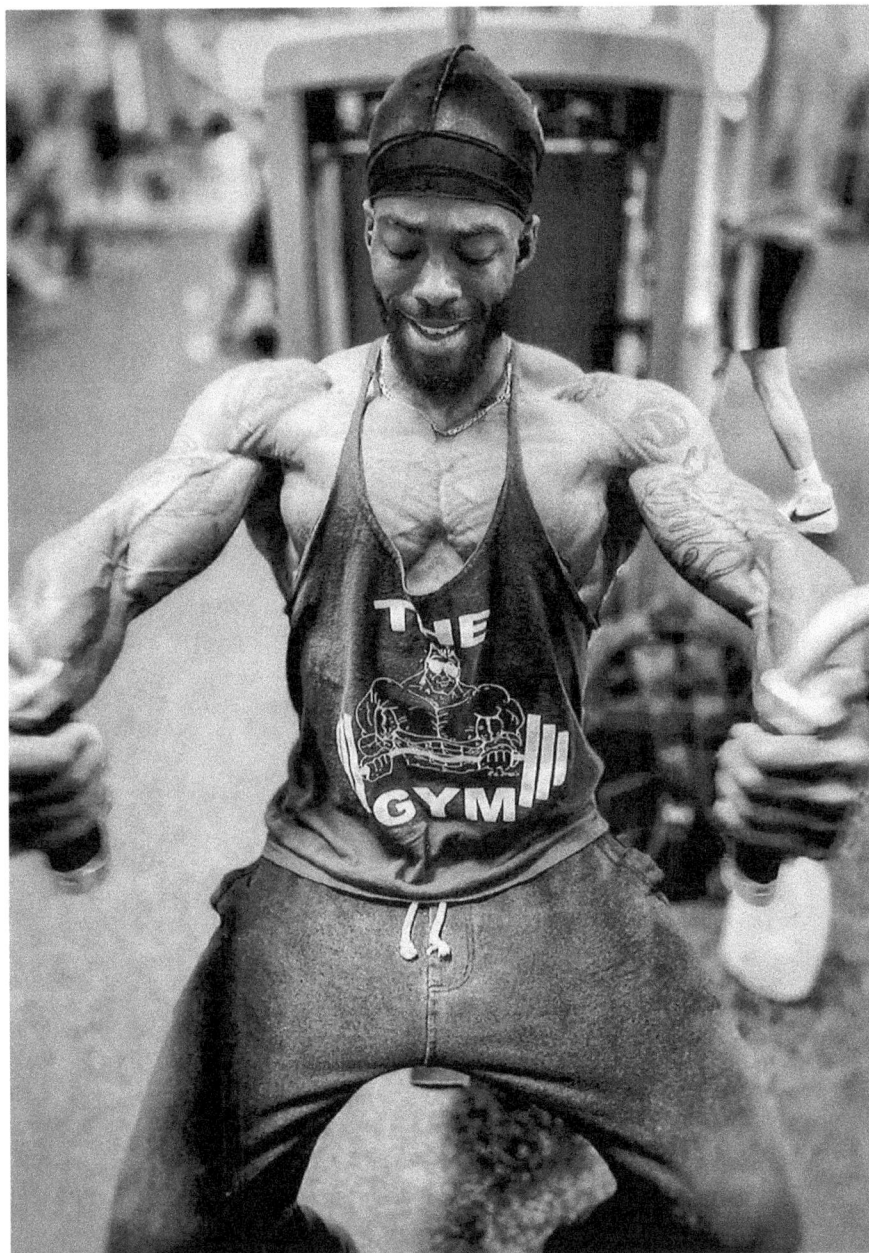

CHEST Fly - Instagram - @djayretroflyy

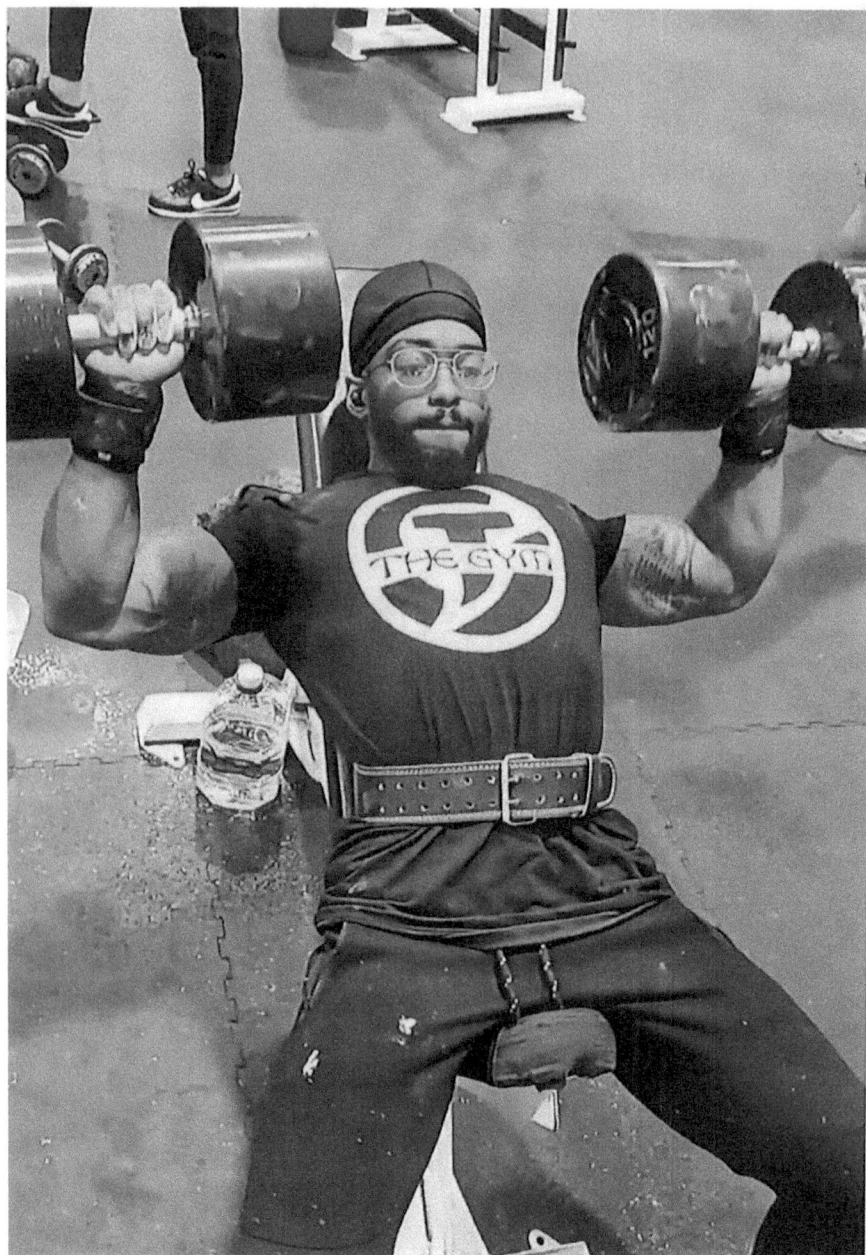

CHEST Incline Dumbbell Press - Instagram - @djayretroflyy

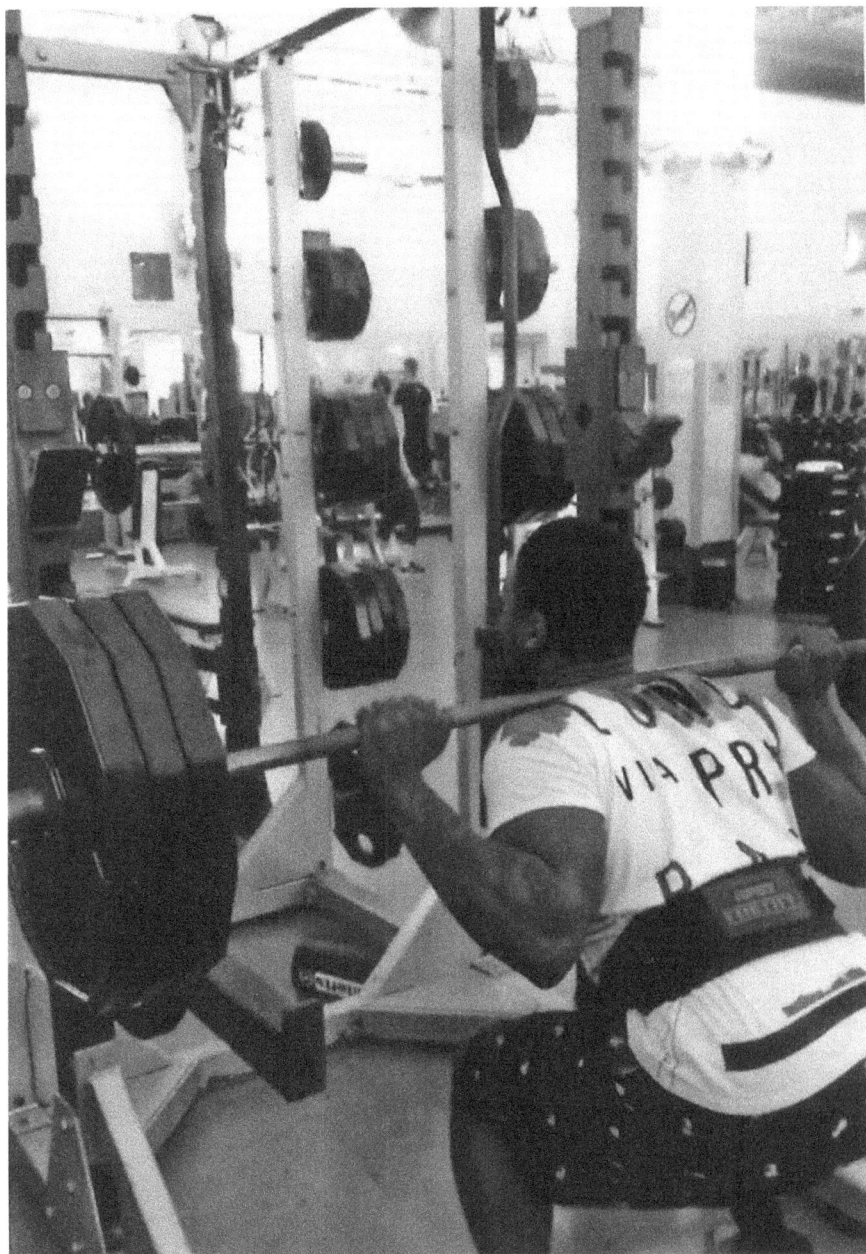

LEGS - Barbell squat

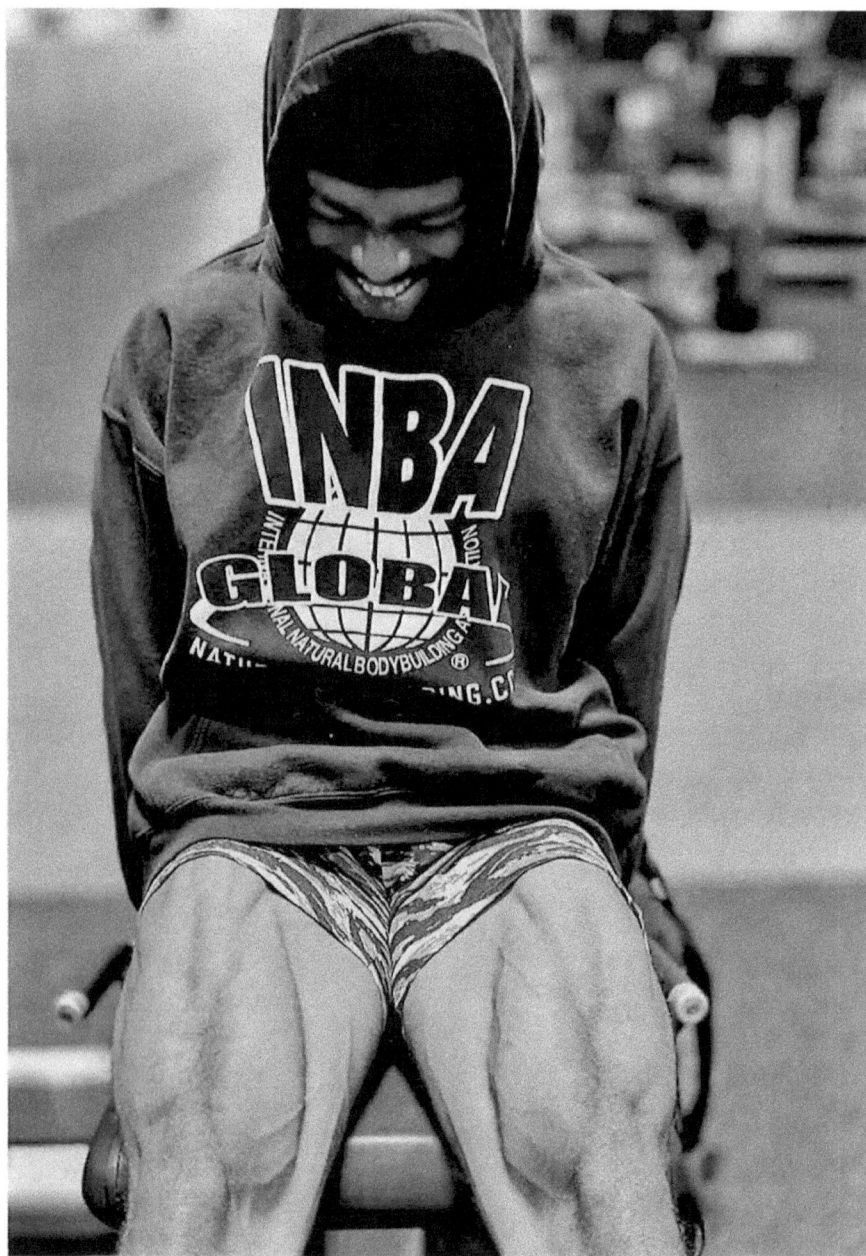

LEGS - Leg Extension

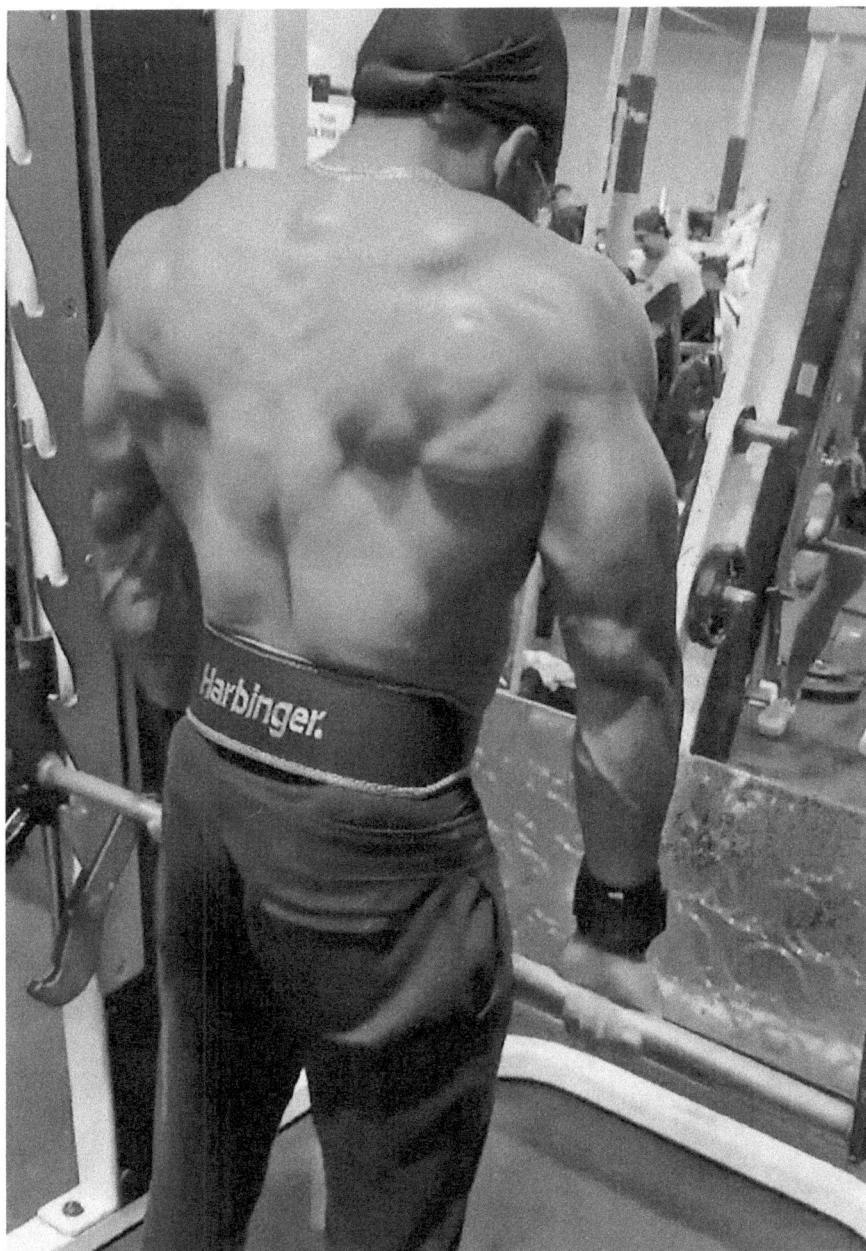

SHOULDERS -Smith Machine Shrugs (Top)

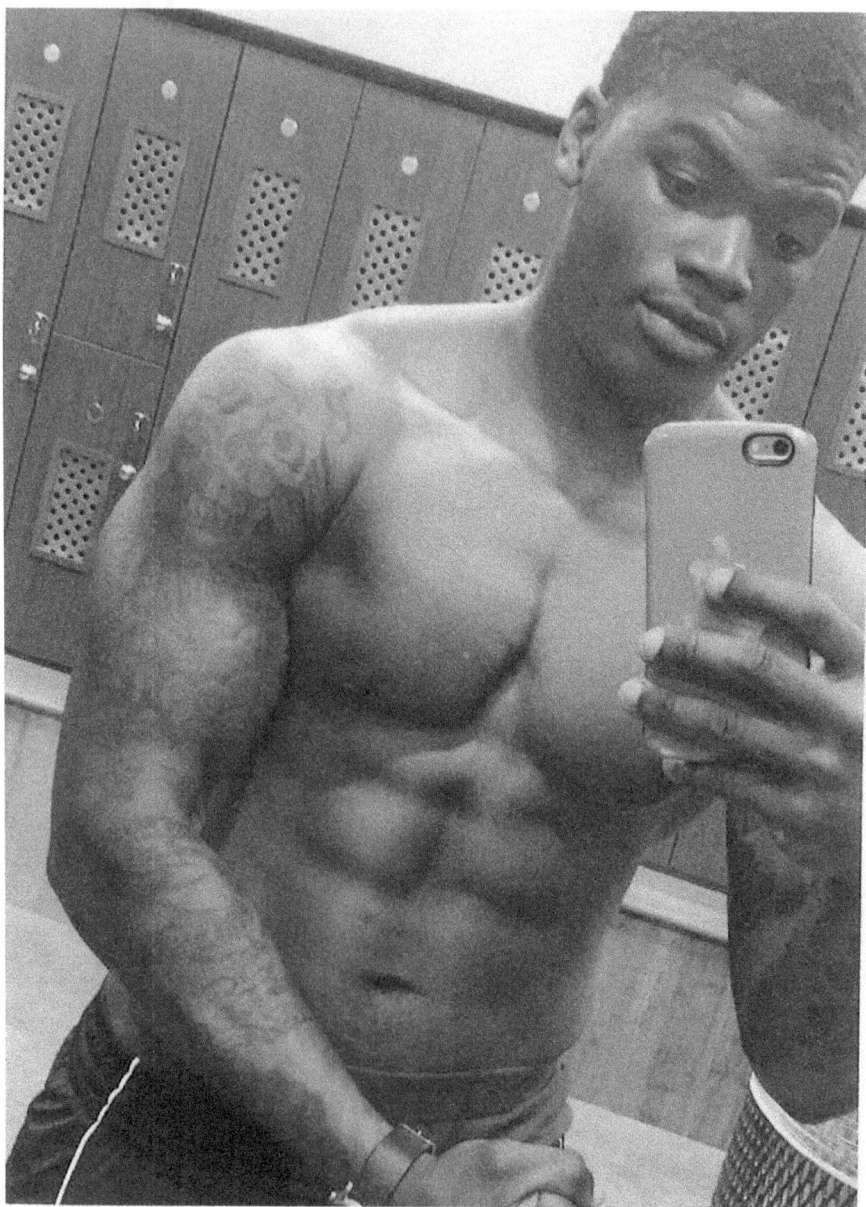

6-WEEK BULK PROGRAM

⬥○〜◦〜○◦⬥

This program is designed to help you increase the number of all of your lifts. A majority of this program consists of compound lifts, which is why the rep range stays low throughout the program. The basis behind this program is that every week, you will increase the weight you've used by 5 to 10 pounds. However, the rep range stays consistent, though you lift heavier each week. If you cannot complete the necessary amount of reps, you will need to break the number of reps down into as few sets as possible until completion.

By the end of week 6, you should not be lifting any less than 30 lbs than you were during week 1. Generally speaking, for those who do not know what weight to begin at, I would recommend starting at 70-75% of your 1RM. For the best results, use 80% of your 1RM.

Contractions are the main focus of this program. Utilize the mind-muscle connection by focusing on the muscle at hand because you are only completing a limited amount of reps. Every time you complete a set, squeeze, and hold that muscle for 5-10 seconds at least twice before going back to complete the next set. Again, 6 weeks is a short period to put on a lot of muscle, but if done correctly, you will notice a significant increase in strength and a change in your body.

NOTES:
DB = Dumbbell
BB = Barbell
W. Grip = Wide Grip

SM = Smith Machine
Good Luck!

EXERCISES	WEEK 1	WEEK 2	WEEK 3	WEEK 4	WEEK 5	WEEK 6
CHEST						
Incline Bench 4x8						
Flat Bench 3x8						
Decline Bench 3x8						
DB Press 3x8						
Peck Deck 3x12						
BACK						
Deadlifts 4x8						
T-Bar Row 4x10						
Lat Pulldown 3x12						

Single Arm DB Row 3x10						
SHOUL-DERS						
Db Shoulder Press 4x8						
BB Military Press 3x8						
Upright Row 3x10						
SM Shrugs 3x10						
Lateral Raises 3x8						
Front Raises 3x8						
ARMS						
BB Curl 4x8						
W. Grip Preacher Curl 3x8						
Dumbbell Curl 4x8						

Skull Crush-ers 3x8						
DB Skull Crushers 3x8						
Tricep Extensions 3x10						

8-WEEK BULK PROGRAM

This program consists of a 5-day split utilizing 6 "abs and touch-ups" as an active rest day. Each phase represents a weekly cycle. Due to this program being accelerated and condensed into 8 weeks, most of the compound lifts may consist of 5 sets. This will allow for a better breakdown of the muscle and more muscle fibers being used, ultimately leading to more growth.

In each phase, you will increase the amount of weight you use and decrease the number of reps. In phase 5, which is the middle of the program, new exercises are introduced in the same scheme to promote muscle confusion and to attack each muscle group from a different angle. Compound moves may stay the same due to it being the most complex movement for that muscle group. The order in which the workouts are done is essential. In the first half of the program, for example, you will be starting off with an incline bench press when doing your chest.

In the second half of the program, you will go from incline to flat, which means that naturally, you will be doing more weight simply by altering the lift's angle. This tactic is methodically planned to help promote heavier lifting without physically trying to tax your body. If your active rest day is too easy, then add a few reps to the ab portion of the workout. Beware of fatiguing the other muscle groups because, as the program continues, the stress would be more strenuous on the muscle.

To put on muscle mass in an 8-week span would require you to have a caloric surplus. Mainly, you would need to increase your protein intake while keeping your fats and, to an extent, your carbohydrates to a minimum. Being that I cannot account for your weight, I would use the statement that "as long as the calories are 'clean', you should take in as much as possible." However, do not excessively eat in one sitting.

You will risk stretching your stomach lining. Break your meals down to 5-6 meals a day.

PHASE 1 – WORKOUT 1: CHEST and BICEPS

WORKOUTS	SETS	REPS	WEIGHT REC-OMMENDED	WEIGHT USED
Incline Bench Press	2/4	12	70% 1RM	
Flat Bench Press	4	12	70% 1RM	
Chest Fly	4	15	Heavy	
Decline DB Press	3	15	65% 10RM	
Standing DB Curl	4	15	Light-Medium	
Concentration Curl	4	15	Light-Medium	

PHASE 1 – WORKOUT 2:   BACK and TRICEPS

WORKOUTS	SETS	REPS	WEIGHT RECOM-MENDED	WEIGHT USED
Dead Lift	2/5	12	70% 1RM	
T-Bar Row	4	12	Light-Medium	
Lat Pull Down ---superset--- Incline DB Row	3 3	15 15	Light-Medium	
Triceps Rope Push Down	4	15	Light-Medium	
DB Skull Crushers	4	15	Light-Medium	

<u>PHASE 1 – WORKOUT 3: SHOULDERS and ABS</u>

WORKOUTS	SETS	REPS	WEIGHT REC-OMMENDED	WEIGHT USED
SM Military Press	2/5	12	70% 10RM	
DB Lateral Raises ---superset---	4	15	Heavy	
Single Arm DB Shoulder Press	4	15	Heavy	
Trap Bar Shrug	4	20	Medium	
DB Front Raises	4	15	Light-Medium	
AB Wheel	4	12		
Crunches	4	20		

PHASE 1 – WORKOUT 4:   ARMS

WORKOUTS	SETS	REPS	WEIGHT REC-OMMENDED	WEIGHT USED
Skull Crushers ---superset--- EZ-Bar Curl	5 5	12 12	Medium Medium	
Incline DB Curls	3	15	Light-Medium	
Triceps Kick-back	3	15	Light-Medium	
DB Preacher Curls ---superset--- DB Hammer Curl	3 3	15 15	Light-Medium Light-Medium	
DB Over Head Triceps Exten-sion	4	15	Light-Medium	

PHASE 1 – WORKOUT 5:   LEGS and TRAPS

WORKOUTS	SETS	REPS	WEIGHT REC-OMMENDED	WEIGHT USED
Squat	2/5	12	70% 1RM	
Front Squat	3	12	Light-Medium	
Leg Curl	4	10	Light-Medium	

Leg Extension	4	10	Light-Medium	
Seated Calf Raises	4	20*	Medium	
Smith Machine Shrugs	4	15	Light-Medium	
Dumbbell Shrugs	4	15	Medium	

PHASE 1 – WORKOUT 6:   ABS and TOUCH-UPS

WORKOUTS	SETS	REPS	WEIGHT RECOMMENDED	WEIGHT USED
Plank	4	45 Sec.		
Sit Ups	4	12	Use Medicine Ball	
Weighted Leg Lift	4	12	10lbs	
DB Forearm Curls	4	15	Heavy	
Barbell Front Raises	4	15	Empty Bar	
Weighted Dips	4	12	Light-Medium	

PHASE 2 – WORKOUT 1:   CHEST and BICEPS

WORKOUTS	SETS	REPS	WEIGHT REC-OMMENDED	WEIGHT USED
Incline Bench Press	2/4	10	75% 1RM	
Flat Bench Press	4	10	75% 1RM	
Chest Fly	4	12	Heavy	
Decline DB Press	3	12	70% 10RM	
Standing DB Curl	4	12	Medium	
Concentration Curl	4	12	Medium	

PHASE 2 – WORKOUT 2:   BACK and TRICEPS

WORKOUTS	SETS	REPS	WEIGHT REC-OMMENDED	WEIGHT USED
Dead Lift	2/5	10	70% 1RM	
T-Bar Row	4	10	Medium	
Lat Pull Down ---superset---	3	12	Medium	
Incline DB Row	3	12	Medium	

Triceps Rope Push Down	4	12	Medium	
DB Skull Crush-ers	4	12	Medium	

PHASE 2 – WORKOUT 3: SHOULDERS and ABS

WORKOUTS	SETS	REPS	WEIGHT REC-OMMENDED	WEIGHT USED
SM Military Press	4	10	75% 10RM	
DB Lateral Raises ---superset---	4	12	Medium-Heavy	
Single Arm DB Shoulder Press	4	12	Medium-Heavy	
Trap Bar Shrug	4	15	Medium-Heavy	
DB Front Raises	3	12	Medium	
AB Wheel	4	15		
Crunches	3	25		

PHASE 2 – WORKOUT 4:   ARMS

WORKOUTS	SETS	REPS	WEIGHT RECOMMENDED	WEIGHT USED
Skull Crushers	5	12	Medium	
---superset--- EZ-Bar Curl	5	12	Medium	
Incline DB Curls	3	15	Light-Medium	
Triceps Kickback	3	15	Light-Medium	
DB Preacher Curls	3	15	Light-Medium	
---superset--- DB Hammer Curl	3	15	Light-Medium	
DB Over Head Triceps Extension	4	15	Light-Medium	

PHASE 2 – WORKOUT 5:   LEGS and TRAPS

WORKOUTS	SETS	REPS	WEIGHT RECOMMENDED	WEIGHT USED
Squat	2/5	10	75% 1RM	
Front Squat	3	10	Medium	
Leg Curl	4	10	Medium	
Leg Extension	4	10	Medium	

Seated Calf Raises	4	15*	Medium-Heavy	
Smith Machine Shrugs	4	12	Medium	
Dumbbell Shrugs	4	12	Medium	

PHASE 2 – WORKOUT 6: ABS and TOUCH-UPS

WORKOUTS	SETS	REPS	WEIGHT REC-OMMENDED	WEIGHT USED
Plank	4	60 Sec.		
Sit Ups	4	15	Use Medicine Ball	
Weighted Leg Lift	4	15	10lbs	
DB Forearm Curls	4	12	Heavy	
Barbell Front Raises	4	12	2.5lbs per side	
Weighted Dips	4	10	Medium	

PHASE 3 – WORKOUT 1:   CHEST and BICEPS

WORKOUTS	SETS	REPS	WEIGHT REC-OMMENDED	WEIGHT USED
Incline Bench Press	2/4	8	80% 1RM	
Flat Bench Press	4	8	80% 1RM	
Chest Fly	4	10	Heavy	
Decline DB Press	3	10	75% 10RM	
Standing DB Curl	4	10	Medium-Heavy	
Concentration Curl	4	10	Medium-Heavy	

PHASE 3 – WORKOUT 2:   BACK and TRICEPS

WORKOUTS	SETS	REPS	WEIGHT REC-OMMENDED	WEIGHT USED
Dead Lift	2/5	8	80% 1RM	
T-Bar Row	4	8	Medium-Heavy	
Lat Pull Down ---superset---	3	10	Medium-Heavy	
Incline DB Row	3	10	Medium-Heavy	
Triceps Rope Push Down	4	10	Medium-Heavy	

DB Skull Crushers	4	10	Medium-Heavy	

PHASE 3 – WORKOUT 3: SHOULDERS and ABS

WORKOUTS	SETS	REPS	WEIGHT RECOMMENDED	WEIGHT USED
SM Military Press	4	8	80% 10RM	
DB Lateral Raises ---superset--- Single Arm DB Shoulder Press	4 4	10 10	Medium-Heavy Medium-Heavy	
Trap Bar Shrug	4	12	Heavy	
DB Front Raises	3	10	Medium-Heavy	
AB Wheel	3	20		
Crunches	4	25		

PHASE 3 – WORKOUT 4:   ARMS

WORKOUTS	SETS	REPS	WEIGHT REC-OMMENDED	WEIGHT USED
Skull Crushers ---superset--- EZ-Bar Curl	5 5	8 8	Medium-Heavy Medium-Heavy	
Incline DB Curls	3	10	Medium-Heavy	
Triceps Kickback	3	10	Medium-Heavy	
DB Preacher Curls ---superset--- DB Hammer Curl	3 3	10 10	Medium-Heavy Medium-Heavy	
DB Over Head Triceps Extension	4	10	Medium-Heavy	

PHASE 3 – WORKOUT 5:   LEGS and TRAPS

WORKOUTS	SETS	REPS	WEIGHT REC-OMMENDED	WEIGHT USED
Squat	2/5	8	80% 1RM	
Front Squat	3	8	Medium-Heavy	
Leg Curl	4	10	Medium-Heavy	
Leg Extension	4	10	Medium-Heavy	
Seated Calf Raises	4	15*	Medium-Heavy	

Smith Machine Shrugs	4	10	Medium-Heavy	
Dumbbell Shrugs	4	10	Medium-Heavy	

PHASE 3 – WORKOUT 6:   ABS and TOUCH-UPS

WORKOUTS	SETS	REPS	WEIGHT REC-OMMENDED	WEIGHT USED
Plank	4	75 Sec.		
Sit Ups	4	20	Use Medicine Ball	
Weighted Leg Lift	4	10	15lbs	
DB Forearm Curls	4	10	Heavy	
Barbell Front Raises	4	10	5lbs per side	
Weighted Dips	4	10	Medium-Heavy	

PHASE 4 – WORKOUT 1:   CHEST and BICEPS

WORKOUTS	SETS	REPS	WEIGHT REC-OMMENDED	WEIGHT USED
Incline Bench Press	2/5	6	80% 1RM	
Flat Bench Press	5	6	80% 1RM	
Chest Fly	4	10	Heavier	
Decline DB Press	3	8	80% 10RM	
Standing DB Curl	4	10	Heavy	
Concentration Curl	4	10	Heavy	

PHASE 4 – WORKOUT 2:   BACK and TRICEPS

WORKOUTS	SETS	REPS	WEIGHT REC-OMMENDED	WEIGHT USED
Dead Lift	2/5	6	80% 1RM	
T-Bar Row	4	8	Heavy	
Lat Pull Down ---superset--- Incline DB Row	3 3	10 10	Heavy Heavy	
Triceps Rope Push Down	4	10	Heavy	

DB Skull Crush-ers	4	8	Heavy	

PHASE 4 – WORKOUT 3: SHOULDERS and ABS

WORKOUTS	SETS	REPS	WEIGHT REC-OMMENDED	WEIGHT USED
SM Military Press	5	6	80% 10RM	
DB Lateral Raises ---superset--- Single Arm DB Shoulder Press	4 4	8 8	Heavy Heavy	
Trap Bar Shrug	4	10	Heavy	
DB Front Raises	3	10	Heavy	
AB Wheel	3	20		
Crunches	4	25		

PHASE 4 – WORKOUT 4:   ARMS

WORKOUTS	SETS	REPS	WEIGHT REC-OMMENDED	WEIGHT USED
Skull Crushers ---superset--- EZ-Bar Curl	5 5	6 6	Heavy Heavy	
Incline DB Curls	3	8	Heavy	
Triceps Kick-back	3	8	Heavy	
DB Preacher Curls ---superset--- DB Hammer Curl	3 3	8 8	Heavy Heavy	
DB Over Head Triceps Extension	4	8	Heavy	

PHASE 4 – WORKOUT 5:   LEGS and TRAPS

WORKOUTS	SETS	REPS	WEIGHT REC-OMMENDED	WEIGHT USED
Squat	2/5	6	85% 1RM	
Front Squat	3	6	Heavy	
Leg Curl	4	8	Heavy	

Leg Extension	4	8	Heavy	
Seated Calf Raises	4	10*	Heavy	
Smith Machine Shrugs	4	10	Heavy	
Dumbbell Shrugs	4	10	Heavy	

PHASE 4 – WORKOUT 6:   ABS and TOUCH-UPS

WORKOUTS	SETS	REPS	WEIGHT RECOMMENDED	WEIGHT USED
Plank	4	90 Sec.		
Sit Ups	3	20	Use Medicine Ball	
Weighted Leg Lift	4	8	20lbs	
DB Forearm Curls	4	10	Heavy	
Barbell Front Raises	4	12	5lbs per side	
Weighted Dips	4	10	Heavy	

PHASE 5 – WORKOUT 1:   CHEST and BICEPS

WORKOUTS	SETS	REPS	WEIGHT REC-OMMENDED	WEIGHT USED
Flat Bench Press	2/4	12	70% 1RM	
Decline Bench Press	4	12	70% 1RM	
Incline Bench Press ***superset*** Incline DB Press	3 3	6 (Lower for 4 sec.) 12	70-75% 1RM 70% 10RM	
Preacher Curl	4	12	Medium	
Concentration Curl	4	12	Medium	

PHASE 5 – WORKOUT 2:   BACK and TRICEPS

WORKOUTS	SETS	REPS	WEIGHT REC-OMMENDED	WEIGHT USED
Dead Lift	2/5	12	70% 1RM	
V-Bar Pull Down	4	12	Medium	
Barbell Row ---superset--- Seated Row	3 3	12 12	70% 10RM Medium	

Triceps Rope Push Down	4	12	Medium	
DB Skull Crushers	4	12	Medium	

PHASE 5 – WORKOUT 3: SHOULDERS and ABS

WORKOUTS	SETS	REPS	WEIGHT REC-OMMENDED	WEIGHT USED
Seated BB Overhead Press	4	12	70% 10RM	
Arnold Presses ---superset--- Single Arm DB Shoulder Press	4 4	12 10	Medium Medium	
Trap Bar Shrug	4	15	Medium	
DB Lateral Raises	4	15	Medium	
AB Wheel	4	12		
Crunches	4	15		

PHASE 5 – WORKOUT 4:   ARMS

WORKOUTS	SETS	REPS	WEIGHT RECOM-MENDED	WEIGHT USED
Close Grip Bench ---superset--- DB Skull Crushers	5 5	10 10	70% 1RM Medium	
Barbell Curl	4	12	Light-Medium	
Skull Crushers	3	15	Light-Medium	
Standing DB Curl ---superset--- Triceps Push Down	3 3	15 15	Medium Medium	
Incline DB Curls	3	12	Medium	

PHASE 5 – WORKOUT 5:   LEGS and TRAPS

WORKOUTS	SETS	REPS	WEIGHT RECOM-MENDED	WEIGHT USED
Squat	2/4	12	70% 1RM	
Leg Press ---superset---	4	15	Medium	
Leg Press Calf Raises	4	15	Medium	
Leg Extension	4	12	Light-Medium	
Leg Curl	4	20*	Medium	
EZ-Bar Upright Row	4	12	Medium	
Dumbbell Shrugs	4	12	Medium	

PHASE 5 – WORKOUT 6:   ABS and TOUCH-UPS

WORKOUTS	SETS	REPS	WEIGHT REC-OMMENDED	WEIGHT USED
Plank	3	90 Sec.		
Sit Ups	3	20	Use Medicine Ball	
Weighted Leg Lift	4	12	5lbs	

BB Forearm Curls	4	15	Heavy	
Barbell Front Raises	4	15	Empty Bar	
Pull Ups	4	12	Body	

PHASE 6 – WORKOUT 1:   CHEST and BICEPS

WORKOUTS	SETS	REPS	WEIGHT REC-OMMENDED	WEIGHT USED
Flat Bench Press	2/4	8	80% 1RM	
Decline Bench Press	4	15	65% 1RM	
Incline Bench Press	3	6 (Lower for 4 sec.)	70-75% 1RM	
superset Incline DB Press	3	10	75% 10RM	
Preacher Curl	4	10	Medium-Heavy	
Concentration Curl	4	10	Medium-Heavy	

PHASE 6 – WORKOUT 2:   BACK and TRICEPS

WORKOUTS	SETS	REPS	WEIGHT REC-OMMENDED	WEIGHT USED
Dead Lift	2/5	10	75% 1RM	
V-Bar Pull Down	4	10	Medium-Heavy	
Barbell Row ---superset--- Seated Row	3 3	10 10	75% 10RM Medium-Heavy	
Ovehead Triceps Extensions	4	10	Medium-Heavy	
DB Kick Backs	4	10	Medium-Heavy	

PHASE 6 – WORKOUT 3:   SHOULDERS and ABS

WORKOUTS	SETS	REPS	WEIGHT REC-OMMENDED	WEIGHT USED
Seated BB Overhead Press	4	10	75% 10RM	
Arnold Presses ---superset--- Single Arm DB Shoulder Press	4 4	10 8	Medium-Heavy Medium-Heavy	
Trap Bar Shrug	4	12	Medium-Heavy	

DB Lateral Raises	4	12	Medium-Heavy	
AB Wheel	4	15		
Crunches	4	10	5lbs	

PHASE 6 – WORKOUT 4: ARMS

WORKOUTS	SETS	REPS	WEIGHT REC-OMMENDED	WEIGHT USED
Close Grip Bench ---superset--- DB Skull Crushers	5 5	8 8	80% 1RM Medium-Heavy	
Barbell Curl	4	10	Medium-Heavy	
Skull Crushers	3	10	Medium-Heavy	
Standing DB Curl ---superset--- Triceps Push Down	3 3	12 12	Medium-Heavy Medium-Heavy	
Incline DB Curls	3	10	Medium-Heavy	

PHASE 6 – WORKOUT 5: LEGS and TRAPS

WORKOUTS	SETS	REPS	WEIGHT REC-OMMENDED	WEIGHT USED
Squat	2/4	10	75% 1RM	
Leg Press ---superset---	4	12	Medium-Heavy	
Leg Press Calf Raises	4	15	Medium-Heavy	
Leg Extension	4	10	Medium-Heavy	
Leg Curl	4	10	Medium-Heavy	
EZ-Bar Upright Row	4	10	Medium-Heavy	
Dumbbell Shrugs	4	10	Heavy	

PHASE 6 – WORKOUT 6: ABS and TOUCH-UPS

WORKOUTS	SETS	REPS	WEIGHT REC-OMMENDED	WEIGHT USED
Plank	4	90 Sec.		
Sit Ups	4	20	Use Medicine Ball	
Weighted Leg Lift	4	8	10lbs	

BB Forearm Curls	4	15	Heavy	
Barbell Front Raises	4	10	5lbs Per Side	
Weighted Pull Ups	4	Failure	25lbs	

PHASE 7 – WORKOUT 1: CHEST and BICEPS

WORKOUTS	SETS	REPS	WEIGHT RECOMMENDED	WEIGHT USED
Flat Bench Press	2/4	6 (Lower for 4 sec.)	85% 1RM	
Decline Bench Press	3	10	75% 1RM	
Incline Bench Press	4	4 (Lower for 3 sec.)	80% 1RM	
superset Incline DB Press	4	8	80% 10RM	
Preacher Curl	4	8	Heavy	
Concentration Curl	4	8	Heavy	

PHASE 7 – WORKOUT 2:   BACK and TRICEPS

WORKOUTS	SETS	REPS	WEIGHT REC-OMMENDED	WEIGHT USED
Dead Lift	2/5	8	80% 1RM	
V-Bar Pull Down	4	8	Heavy	
Barbell Row ---superset--- Seated Row	3 3	8 8	80% 10RM Heavy	
Overhead Triceps Extensions	4	8	Heavy	
DB Kick Backs	4	8	Heavy	

PHASE 7 – WORKOUT 3:   SHOULDERS and ABS

WORKOUTS	SETS	REPS	WEIGHT REC-OMMENDED	WEIGHT USED
Seated BB Overhead Press	4	8	80% 10RM	
Arnold Presses ---superset--- Single Arm DB Shoulder Press	4 4	8 6	Heavy Heavy	
Trap Bar Shrug	4	8	Heavy	

DB Lateral Raises	4	8	Heavy	
AB Wheel	4	20		
Weighted Leg Lift	4	10	10lbs	

PHASE 7 – WORKOUT 4:   ARMS

WORKOUTS	SETS	REPS	WEIGHT RECOMMENDED	WEIGHT USED
Close Grip Bench ---superset--- DB Skull Crushers	5 5	6 6	85% 1RM Heavy	
Barbell Curl	4	6	Heavy	
Skull Crushers	3	8	Heavy	
Standing DB Curl ---superset--- Triceps Push Down	3 3	10 10	Heavy Heavy	
Incline DB Curls	3	8	Heavy	

PHASE 7 – WORKOUT 5: LEGS and TRAPS

WORKOUTS	SETS	REPS	WEIGHT REC-OMMENDED	WEIGHT USED
Squat	2/4	8	80% 1RM	
Leg Press ---superset--- Leg Press Calf Raises	4 4	10 12	Heavy Heavy	
Leg Extension	4	8	Heavy	
Leg Curl	4	8	Heavy	
EZ-Bar Upright Row	4	8	Heavy	
Dumbbell Shrugs	4	8	Heavy	

PHASE 7 – WORKOUT 6: ABS and TOUCH-UPS

WORKOUTS	SETS	REPS	WEIGHT REC-OMMENDED	WEIGHT USED
Plank	4	90 Sec.		
Sit Ups	4	25	Use Medicine Ball	
Weighted Leg Lift	4	6	15lbs	

BB Forearm Curls	4	15	Heavy	
Barbell Front Raises	4	8	7.5lbs Per Side	
Weighted Pull Ups	4	Failure	35lbs	

PHASE 8 – WORKOUT 1:   CHEST and BICEPS

WORKOUTS	SETS	REPS	WEIGHT REC-OMMENDED	WEIGHT USED
Flat Bench Press	2/5	5 (Lower for 4 sec.)	90% 1RM	
Decline Bench Press	3	6	75% 1RM	
Incline Bench Press	5	4 (Lower for 3 sec.)	80% 1RM	
superset Incline DB Press	5	5	90% 10RM	
Preacher Curl	5	6	Heavy	
Concentration Curl	5	6	Heavy	

PHASE 8 – WORKOUT 2:   BACK and TRICEPS

WORKOUTS	SETS	REPS	WEIGHT REC-OMMENDED	WEIGHT USED
Dead Lift	2/6	6	85% 1RM	
V-Bar Pull Down	4	8	Heavy	
Barbell Row ---superset--- Seated Row	4 4	8 8	80% 10RM Heavy	
Overhead Triceps Extensions	4	10	Heavy	
DB Kick Backs	4	10	Heavy	

PHASE 8 – WORKOUT 3:   SHOULDERS and ABS

WORKOUTS	SETS	REPS	WEIGHT REC-OMMENDED	WEIGHT USED
Seated BB Overhead Press	4	6	85% 10RM	
Arnold Presses ---superset--- Single Arm DB Shoulder Press	4 4	6 6	Heavy Heavy	
Trap Bar Shrug	5	8	Heavy	

DB Lateral Raises	5	8	Heavy	
AB Wheel	4	20		
Weighted Leg Lift	4	10	15lbs	

PHASE 8 – WORKOUT 4:   ARMS

WORKOUTS	SETS	REPS	WEIGHT REC-OMMENDED	WEIGHT USED
Close Grip Bench ---superset--- DB Skull Crushers	6 6	6 6	85% 1RM Heavy	
Barbell Curl	3	8	Heavy	
Skull Crushers	4	8	Heavy	
Standing DB Curl ---superset--- Triceps Push Down	4 4	8 8	Heavy Heavy	
Incline DB Curls	4	8	Heavy	

PHASE 8 – WORKOUT 5: LEGS and TRAPS

WORKOUTS	SETS	REPS	WEIGHT REC-OMMENDED	WEIGHT USED
Squat	2/5	6	85% 1RM	
Leg Press ---superset--- Leg Press Calf Raises	5 5	8 10	Heavy Heavy	
Leg Extension	3	12	Heavy	
Leg Curl	3	12	Heavy	
EZ-Bar Upright Row	4	8	Heavy	
Dumbbell Shrugs	4	8	Heavy	

PHASE 8 – WORKOUT 6: ABS and TOUCH-UPS

WORKOUTS	SETS	REPS	WEIGHT REC-OMMENDED	WEIGHT USED
Plank	5	90 Sec.		
Sit Ups	4	25	Use Medicine Ball	
Weighted Leg Lift	4	6	20lbs	

BB Forearm Curls	4	12	Heavy	
Barbell Front Raises	4	8	10lbs Per Side	
Weighted Pull Ups	4	Failure	45lbs	

8 WEEK SHRED PROGRAM

This program is based on a 5-day split but incorporates one extra day, which is designed for a full-body exercise. Due to the program's condensed nature, a cardio regimen is added to accelerate fat burning. 8 weeks is a short period of time to fully explore the evolution of shredding body fat without sacrificing muscular development, however, this program utilizes heavy cardiovascular mobility to assist in dropping the pounds off rapidly. Every other day, you will be required to do a cardio exercise of your choice. Beginning at 15 minutes, you will add 1 minute to your cardio sessions until the completion of the program.

This program is broken down into 8 phases, each phase representing one week. Though the reps change, the workouts throughout the program stay consistent until phase 5, which is the halfway point of the program where new exercises are introduced. A training split is used to isolate each muscle group for specific targeting. Each exercise begins with a heavy compound movement. Each week, you will increase the weight of this lift and lower the repetitions. Each other accompanying lift will consist of the opposite approach. You will lower the weight but complete more repetitions. By phase 5, your body should be in a good state of conditioning which then would require you to amplify the intensity of the workouts by increasing the total volume of the exercise.

Lastly, a major part of the shredding phase will also consist of better eating habits. Because I am not certain of your caloric intake daily, nor do

I know how many pounds you are trying to lose, I will provide a general guideline to amplify your results.

Phase 1 – Monitor your eating after your last meal of the day; if possible, try to resolve not to eat after 9 pm.

Phase 2 – At this point, you should be pulling back from heavy carbs such as bread, cakes, cookies, and pasta as well as heavy fat items such as pork products and foods containing high sugars like candy and cereal.

Phase 3 – At this phase, you should not be consuming food after 8:30 pm. Lower your daily calorie count by 250 calories.

Phase 4 – Introduce calorie supplementation by using a gallon of water daily. This will help you curve your hunger.

Phase 5 – Consume all carbs prior to your workout. If you work out early in the day, then try to keep your carb intake to a minimum post-workout. Also, eliminate bread and heavy starch items completely.

Phase 6 – Decrease calorie count by another 250 calories. By this point, your body will be accustomed to cardio, so take advantage of this by eating as clean as possible.

Phase 7 – Keep pushing! Try to consume all meals before 8 pm. Increase water intake to 1 ½ gallons per day. Lower your carbs pre-workout.

Phase 8 – The last week, you will complete a peak phase, which will consist of carb loading. You will intake simple carbs such as oatmeal and rice to reach your carb count. Also, keep fats to a minimum.

PHASE 1 – WORKOUT 1: CHEST and ABS (Lower)

WORKOUTS	SETS	REPS	WEIGHT RECOMMENDED	WEIGHT USED
Incline Bench Press	2/4	12*	70% 1RM	
Decline Dumbbell Press	3	10	75% 10RM	
Chest Fly	4	10	Heavy	

Push Ups	3	Failure	30-Second Breaks	
Dumbbell Press (Flat Bench)	3	8*	80% 10RM	
Leg Kick Outs	4	12	N/A	
Hanging Leg Raises	4	12	Body Weight	

PHASE 1 – WORKOUT 2: BACK and 15 Minutes Cardio

WORKOUTS	SETS	REPS	WEIGHT RECOMMENDED	WEIGHT USED
Barbell Row	4	12*	70% 10RM	
Lat Pulldown	4	10	Medium-Heavy	
Seated Row	3	10	75% 10RM	
Pull Ups	3	Failure	30-Second Breaks	
Bent Over Dumbbell Flys	3	10*	Heavy	
15 Minutes PACED Cardio				

PHASE 1 – WORKOUT 3: SHOULDERS and ABS (Obliques)

WORKOUTS	SETS	REPS	WEIGHT REC-OMMENDED	WEIGHT USED
SM Military Press	4	12	70% 10RM	
DB Lateral Raises	3	10	Heavy	
DB Front Raises	3	10	Heavy	
SM Shrugs	4	10*	Heavy	
Single Arm DB Shoulder Press	3	10	70% 10RM	
Russian Twist	4	12	Body	
Standing DB Oblique Crunch	4	12	Heavy	

PHASE 1 – WORKOUT 4: ARMS and 16 Minutes Cardio

WORKOUTS	SETS	REPS	WEIGHT REC-OMMENDED	WEIGHT USED
Skull Crushers	4	12	Medium	
Preacher Curl	4	10	Heavy	
Triceps Cable Pushdown	4	10	Medium-Heavy	
Lying DB Extensions	3	10	Medium-Heavy	
Incline DB Curls	3	10	Medium-Heavy	
DB Hammer Curl	3	10	Heavy	
16 Minutes PACED Cardio				

PHASE 1 – WORKOUT 5: LEGS and ABS (Mid/Top)

WORKOUTS	SETS	REPS	WEIGHT REC-OMMENDED	WEIGHT USED
Squat	2/5	12	70% 1RM	
Straight Leg Dead Lifts	3	12	Heavy	
Leg Extensions	4	10	Medium-Heavy	
Leg Curl	4	10	Medium-Heavy	
Seated Calf Raises	4	12*	Heavy	
Toe Touches	4	12		
Crunches	4	20		

PHASE 1 – WORKOUT 6: FULL BODY and 17 Minutes Cardio

WORKOUTS	SETS	REPS	WEIGHT REC-OMMENDED	WEIGHT USED
Dead Lift	2/4	12	70% 1RM	
Leg Press	4	10	Heavy	
Close Grip Bench Press	4	10	70% 10RM	

Single Arm DB Row	4	10	Heavy	
Rear Delt Flys	4	10	Medium-Heavy	
17-Minute PACED Cardio				

PHASE 2 – WORKOUT 1: CHEST and ABS (Lower)

WORKOUTS	SETS	REPS	WEIGHT RECOMMENDED	WEIGHT USED
Incline Bench Press	2/4	10*	75% 1RM	
Decline Dumbbell Press	3	12	70% 10RM	
Chest Fly	4	10	Medium-Heavy	
Push Ups	3	Failure	25-Second Breaks	
Dumbbell Press (Flat Bench)	3	12*	70% 10RM	
Leg Kick Outs	4	15	N/A	
Hanging Leg Raises	4	15	Body Weight	

PHASE 2 – WORKOUT 2: BACK and 18 Minutes Cardio

WORKOUTS	SETS	REPS	WEIGHT REC-OMMENDED	WEIGHT USED
Barbell Row	4	10*	75% 10RM	
Lat Pulldown	4	12	Medium-Heavy	
Seated Row	3	12	70% 10RM	
Pull Ups	3	Failure	25-Second Breaks	
Bent Over Dumbbell Flys	3	10*	Heavy	
18 Minutes PACED Cardio				

PHASE 2 – WORKOUT 3: SHOULDERS and ABS (Obliques)

WORKOUTS	SETS	REPS	WEIGHT REC-OMMENDED	WEIGHT USED
SM Military Press	4	12	70% 10RM	
DB Lateral Raises	3	12	Medium-Heavy	
DB Front Raises	3	12	Medium-Heavy	
SM Shrugs	4	12*	Medium-Heavy	

Single Arm DB Shoulder Press	3	12	65% 10RM	
Russian Twist	4	15	Body	
Standing DB Oblique Crunch	4	15	Medium-Heavy	

PHASE 2 – WORKOUT 4: ARMS and 19 Minutes Cardio

WORKOUTS	SETS	REPS	WEIGHT RECOMMENDED	WEIGHT USED
Skull Crushers	4	10	Medium-Heavy	
Preacher Curl	4	12	Medium-Heavy	
Triceps Cable Pushdown	4	12	Medium	
Lying DB Extensions	3	12	Medium	
Incline DB Curls	3	12	Medium	
DB Hammer Curl	3	12	Medium-Heavy	
19 Minutes PACED Cardio				

PHASE 2 – WORKOUT 5: LEGS and ABS (Mid/Top)

WORKOUTS	SETS	REPS	WEIGHT RECOMMENDED	WEIGHT USED
Squat	2/5	10	75% 1RM	
Straight Leg Dead Lifts	3	12	Medium-Heavy	
Leg Extensions	4	12	Medium	
Leg Curl	4	12	Medium	
Seated Calf Raises	4	15*	Medium-Heavy	
Toe Touches	4	12		
Crunches	3	35		

PHASE 2 – WORKOUT 6: FULL BODY and 20 Minutes Cardio

WORKOUTS	SETS	REPS	WEIGHT RECOMMENDED	WEIGHT USED
Dead Lift	2/4	10	75% 1RM	
Leg Press	4	12	Medium-Heavy	
Close Grip Bench Press	4	12	70% 10RM	

Single Arm DB Row	4	12	Medium-Heavy	
Rear Delt Flys	4	12	Medium	
20-Minute PACED Cardio				

PHASE 3 – WORKOUT 1: CHEST and ABS (Lower)

WORKOUTS	SETS	REPS	WEIGHT RECOMMENDED	WEIGHT USED
Incline Bench Press	2/4	8*	80% 1RM	
Decline Dumbbell Press	3	15	65% 10RM	
Chest Fly	4	12	Medium	
Push Ups	3	Failure	20-Second Breaks	
Dumbbell Press (Flat Bench)	3	15*	65% 10RM	
Leg Kick Outs	4	20	N/A	
Hanging Leg Raises	3	20	Body Weight	

PHASE 3 – WORKOUT 2: BACK and 21 Minutes Cardio

WORKOUTS	SETS	REPS	WEIGHT REC-OMMENDED	WEIGHT USED
Barbell Row	4	8*	80% 10RM	
Lat Pulldown	4	15	Medium	
Seated Row	3	15	65% 10RM	
Pull Ups	3	Failure	20-Second Breaks	
Bent Over Dumbbell Flys	3	15*	Medium	
21 Minutes PACED Cardio				

PHASE 3 – WORKOUT 3: SHOULDERS and ABS (Obliques)

WORKOUTS	SETS	REPS	WEIGHT REC-OMMENDED	WEIGHT USED
SM Military Press	4	10	70% 10RM	
DB Lateral Raises	3	15	Medium-Heavy	
DB Front Raises	3	15	Medium-Heavy	

SM Shrugs	4	15*	Medium-Heavy	
Single Arm DB Shoulder Press	3	15	65% 10RM	
Russian Twist	4	20	Body	
Standing DB Oblique Crunch	4	20	Medium-Heavy	

PHASE 3 – WORKOUT 4: ARMS and 22 Minutes Cardio

WORKOUTS	SETS	REPS	WEIGHT REC-OMMENDED	WEIGHT USED
Skull Crushers	4	8	Heavy	
Preacher Curl	4	15	Medium	
Triceps Cable Pushdown	4	15	Light-Medium	
Lying DB Extensions	3	15	Light-Medium	
Incline DB Curls	3	15	Light-Medium	
DB Hammer Curl	3	15	Medium	

22 Minutes PACED Cardio				

PHASE 3 – WORKOUT 5: LEGS and ABS (Mid/Top)

WORKOUTS	SETS	REPS	WEIGHT RECOMMENDED	WEIGHT USED
Squat	2/5	8	80% 1RM	
Straight Leg Dead Lifts	3	15	Medium	
Leg Extensions	4	15	Medium	
Leg Curl	4	15	Medium	
Seated Calf Raises	4	15*	Medium-Heavy	
Toe Touches	4	20		
Crunches	3	50		

PHASE 3 – WORKOUT 6: FULL BODY and 23 Minutes Cardio

WORKOUTS	SETS	REPS	WEIGHT REC-OMMENDED	WEIGHT USED
Dead Lift	2/4	10	75% 1RM	
Leg Press	4	12	Medium-Heavy	
Close Grip Bench Press	4	12	70% 10RM	
Single Arm DB Row	4	12	Medium-Heavy	
Rear Delt Flys	4	12	Medium	
23-Minute PACED Cardio				

PHASE 4 – WORKOUT 1: CHEST and ABS (Lower)

WORKOUTS	SETS	REPS	WEIGHT REC-OMMENDED	WEIGHT USED
Incline Bench Press	2/4	6*	85% 1RM	
Decline Dumbbell Press	3	20	55-60% 10RM	
Chest Fly	4	15	Light-Medium	

Push Ups	3	Failure	15-Second Breaks	
Dumbbell Press (Flat Bench)	3	20*	55-60% 10RM	
Leg Kick Outs	4	30	N/A	
Hanging Leg Raises	3	25	Body Weight	

PHASE 4 – WORKOUT 2: BACK and 24 Minutes Cardio

WORKOUTS	SETS	REPS	WEIGHT REC-OMMENDED	WEIGHT USED
Barbell Row	4	6*	85% 10RM	
Lat Pulldown	4	20	Light-Medium	
Seated Row	3	20	55-60% 10RM	
Pull Ups	3	Failure	15-Second Breaks	
Bent Over Dumbbell Flys	3	20*	Light-Medium	
24 Minutes PACED Cardio				

PHASE 4 – WORKOUT 3: SHOULDERS and ABS (Obliques)

WORKOUTS	SETS	REPS	WEIGHT REC-OMMENDED	WEIGHT USED
SM Military Press	4	8	80% 10RM	
DB Lateral Raises	3	20	Light-Medium	
DB Front Raises	3	20	Light-Medium	

SM Shrugs	4	20*	Light-Medium	
Single Arm DB Shoulder Press	3	20	55-60% 10RM	
Russian Twist	4	25	Body	
Standing DB Oblique Crunch	4	25	Light-Medium	

PHASE 4 – WORKOUT 4: ARMS and 25 Minutes Cardio

WORKOUTS	SETS	REPS	WEIGHT RECOMMENDED	WEIGHT USED
Skull Crushers	4	15	Medium	
Preacher Curl	4	20	Light-Medium	
Triceps Cable Pushdown	4	20	Light-Medium	
Lying DB Extensions	3	20	Light-Medium	
Incline DB Curls	3	20	Light-Medium	
DB Hammer Curl	3	20	Light-Medium	
25 Minutes PACED Cardio				

PHASE 4 – WORKOUT 5: LEGS and ABS (Mid/Top)

WORKOUTS	SETS	REPS	WEIGHT REC-OMMENDED	WEIGHT USED
Squat	2/5	6	85% 1RM	
Straight Leg Dead Lifts	3	20	Light-Medium	
Leg Exten-sions	4	20	Light-Medium	
Leg Curl	4	20	Light-Medium	
Seated Calf Raises	4	20*	Medium	
Toe Touches	4	25		
Crunches	3	50		

PHASE 4 – WORKOUT 6: FULL BODY and 26 Minutes Cardio

WORKOUTS	SETS	REPS	WEIGHT REC- OMMENDED	WEIGHT USED
Dead Lift	2/4	6	85% 1RM	
Leg Press	4	20	Light-Medium	
Close Grip Bench Press	4	20	55-60% 10RM	
Single Arm DB Row	4	20	Light-Medium	
Rear Delt Flys	4	20	Light-Medium	
26-Minute PACED Cardio				

PHASE 5 – WORKOUT 1: CHEST and ABS (Lower)

WORKOUTS	SETS	REPS	WEIGHT REC-OMMENDED	WEIGHT USED
Flat Bench Press	2/4	12*	70% 1RM	
Single Arm Incline DB Press	4	10	75% 10RM	
Decline SM Press	4	10	Heavy	
Dips	3	Failure	30-Second Breaks	
Dumbbell Fly (Flat Bench)	3	8*	80% 10RM	
Leg Kick Outs	4	12	N/A	
Hanging Leg Raises	4	12	Body Weight	

PHASE 5 – WORKOUT 2: BACK and 27 Minutes Cardio

WORKOUTS	SETS	REPS	WEIGHT RECOMMENDED	WEIGHT USED
Dead Lift	2/4	12*	70% 1RM	
Reverse Grip Pull Down	4	10	Medium-Heavy	
Seated Row	3	10	75% 10RM	
Chin Ups	3	Failure	30-Second Breaks	
Single Arm DB Row	3	10*	Heavy	
27 Minutes PACED Cardio				

PHASE 5 – WORKOUT 3: SHOULDERS and ABS (Obliques)

WORKOUTS	SETS	REPS	WEIGHT RECOMMENDED	WEIGHT USED
SM Behind Neck Press	4	12	70% 10RM	
DB Arnold Press	3	10	Heavy	
Trap Bar Shrug	3	10	Heavy	

Lateral Raises	4	10*	Heavy	
Front Raises	3	10	Heavy	
Russian Twist	4	12	Body	
Standing DB Oblique Crunch	4	12	Heavy	

PHASE 5 – WORKOUT 4: ARMS and 28 Minutes Cardio

WORKOUTS	SETS	REPS	WEIGHT RECOMMENDED	WEIGHT USED
Close Grip Bench Press	4	12	Medium	
Barbell Curl	4	10	Heavy	
Triceps Cable Pushdown	4	10	Heavy	
DB Kickbacks	3	10	Heavy	
Standing Dumb-bell Curls	3	10	Heavy	
Concentration Curl	3	10	Heavy	

28 Minutes PACED Cardio				

PHASE 5 – WORKOUT 5: LEGS and ABS (Mid/Top)

WORKOUTS	SETS	REPS	WEIGHT RECOMMENDED	WEIGHT USED
Leg Press	2/5	12	70% 10RM	
Dumbbell Lunge	3	12	Heavy	
Goblet Squat	4	10	Heavy	
SM Calf Raises	4	10	Heavy	
Leg Curls	4	12*	Heavy	
Toe Touches	4	12		
Crunches	4	20		

PHASE 5 – WORKOUT 6: FULL BODY and 29 Minutes Cardio

WORKOUTS	SETS	REPS	WEIGHT REC-OMMENDED	WEIGHT USED
Barbell Row (Underhand Grip)	4	12	70% 10RM	
---superset--- Rear Delt Fly	4	10	Heavy	
Decline Bench Press	4	10	75% 1RM	
Leg Extensions	4	10	Heavy	
Upright Row (EZ-Bar)	4	10	Heavy	
29-Minute PACED Cardio				

PHASE 6 – WORKOUT 1: CHEST and ABS (Lower)

WORKOUTS	SETS	REPS	WEIGHT REC-OMMENDED	WEIGHT USED
Flat Bench Press	2/4	10*	75% 1RM	
Single Arm Incline DB Press	3	15	65% 10RM	
Decline SM Press	4	15	Medium	
Dips	3	Failure	25-Second Breaks	
Dumbbell Fly (Flat Bench)	3	15*	65% 10RM	
Leg Kick Outs	4	20	N/A	
Hanging Leg Raises	4	20	Body Weight	

PHASE 6 – WORKOUT 2: BACK and 30 Minutes Cardio

WORKOUTS	SETS	REPS	WEIGHT REC-OMMENDED	WEIGHT USED
Dead Lift	4	10*	75% 1RM	
Reverse Grip Pull Down	4	15	Medium	
Seated Row	3	15	65% 10RM	
Chin Ups	3	Failure	25-Second Breaks	
Single Arm DB Row	3	15*	Medium	
30 Minutes PACED Cardio				

PHASE 6 – WORKOUT 3: SHOULDERS and ABS (Obliques)

WORKOUTS	SETS	REPS	WEIGHT REC-OMMENDED	WEIGHT USED
SM Behind Neck Press	4	12	70% 10RM	
DB Arnold Press	3	15	Medium	
Trap Bar Shrug	3	15	Medium	

Lateral Raises	4	15*	Medium	
Front Raises	3	15	65% 10RM	
Russian Twist	4	20	Body	
Standing DB Oblique Crunch	4	20	Medium	

PHASE 6 – WORKOUT 4: ARMS and 31 Minutes Cardio

WORKOUTS	SETS	REPS	WEIGHT REC-OMMENDED	WEIGHT USED
Close Grip Bench Press	4	10	Medium-Heavy	
Barbell Curl	4	15	Medium	
Triceps Cable Pushdown	4	15	Medium	
DB Kickbacks	3	15	Medium	
Standing Dumbbell Curls	3	15	Medium	
Concentration Curl	3	15	Medium	

31 Minutes PACED Cardio				

PHASE 6 – WORKOUT 5: LEGS and ABS (Mid/Top)

WORKOUTS	SETS	REPS	WEIGHT RECOMMENDED	WEIGHT USED
Leg Press	2/5	10	75% 10RM	
Dumbbell Lunge	3	15	Medium	
Goblet Squat	4	15	Medium	
SM Calf Raises	4	15	Medium	
Leg Curls	4	15*	Medium	
Toe Touches	4	12		
Crunches	3	35		

PHASE 6 – WORKOUT 6: FULL BODY and 32 Minutes Cardio

WORKOUTS	SETS	REPS	WEIGHT REC-OMMENDED	WEIGHT USED
Barbell Row (underhand grip)	2/4	10	75% 10RM	
---superset--- Rear Delt Fly	4	15	Medium	
Decline Bench Press	4	15	65% 1RM	
Leg Extensions	4	15	Medium	
Upright Row (EZ-Bar)	4	15	Medium	
32-Minute PACED Cardio				

PHASE 7 – WORKOUT 1: CHEST and ABS (Lower)

WORKOUTS	SETS	REPS	WEIGHT REC-OMMENDED	WEIGHT USED
Flat Bench Press	2/4	8*	80% 1RM	
Single Arm Incline DB Press	3	20	55-60% 10RM	
Decline SM Press	4	20	Light-Medium	
Dips	3	Failure	20-Second Breaks	
Dumbbell Fly (Flat Bench)	3	20*	55-60% 10RM	
Leg Kick Outs	4	25	N/A	
Hanging Leg Raises	3	25	Body Weight	

PHASE 7 – WORKOUT 2: BACK and 33 Minutes Cardio

WORKOUTS	SETS	REPS	WEIGHT REC-OMMENDED	WEIGHT USED
Dead Lift	4	8*	80% 1RM	
Reverse Grip Pull Down	4	20	Light-Medium	
Seated Row	3	20	55-60% 10RM	
Chin Ups	3	Failure	20-Second Breaks	
Single Arm DB Row	3	30*	Light-Medium	
33 Minutes PACED Cardio				

PHASE 7 – WORKOUT 3: SHOULDERS and ABS (Obliques)

WORKOUTS	SETS	REPS	WEIGHT REC-OMMENDED	WEIGHT USED
SM Behind Neck Press	4	10	75% 10RM	
DB Arnold Press	3	20	Light-Medium	
Trap Bar Shrug	3	20	Light-Medium	

Lateral Raises	4	20*	Light-Medium	
Front Raises	3	20	55-60% 10RM	
Russian Twist	4	25	Body	
Standing DB Oblique Crunch	4	25	Light-Medium	

PHASE 7 – WORKOUT 4: ARMS and 34 Minutes Cardio

WORKOUTS	SETS	REPS	WEIGHT REC-OMMENDED	WEIGHT USED
Close Grip Bench Press	4	8	Heavy	
Barbell Curl	4	20	Light	
Triceps Cable Pushdown	4	20	Light-Medium	
DB Kickbacks	3	20	Light-Medium	
Standing Dumbbell Curls	3	20	Light-Medium	
Concentration Curl	3	20	Light-Medium	

34 Minutes PACED Cardio				

PHASE 7 – WORKOUT 5: LEGS and ABS (Mid/Top)

WORKOUTS	SETS	REPS	WEIGHT RECOMMENDED	WEIGHT USED
Leg Press	2/5	8	80% 10RM	
Dumbbell Lunge	3	20	Light-Medium	
Goblet Squat	4	20	Light-Medium	
SM Calf Raises	4	20	Light-Medium	
Leg Curls	4	20*	Medium	
Toe Touches	4	25		
Crunches	3	50		

PHASE 7 – WORKOUT 6: FULL BODY and 35 Minutes Cardio

WORKOUTS	SETS	REPS	WEIGHT REC-OMMENDED	WEIGHT USED
Barbell Row (underhand grip)	2/4	8	80% 10RM	
---superset--- Rear Delt Fly	4	20	Light-Medium	
Decline Bench Press	4	20	65% 1RM	
Leg Extensions	4	20	Medium	
Upright Row (EZ-Bar)	4	20	Medium	
35-Minute PACED Cardio				

PHASE 8 – WORKOUT 1: CHEST and ABS (Lower)

WORKOUTS	SETS	REPS	WEIGHT REC-OMMENDED	WEIGHT USED
Flat Bench Press	2/4	6*	85% 1RM	
Single Arm Incline DB Press	3	25	50-55% 10RM	
Decline SM Press	4	25	Light	
Dips	3	Failure	15-Second Breaks	
Dumbbell Fly (Flat Bench)	3	25*	55-60% 10RM	
Leg Kick Outs	4	30	N/A	
Hanging Leg Raises	3	25	Body Weight	

PHASE 8 – WORKOUT 2: BACK and 36 Minutes Cardio

WORKOUTS	SETS	REPS	WEIGHT REC-OMMENDED	WEIGHT USED
Dead Lift	4	6*	85% 1RM	
Reverse Grip Pull Down	4	25	Light-Medium	
Seated Row	3	25	50-55% 10RM	
Chin Ups	3	Failure	15-Second Breaks	
Single Arm DB Row	3	25*	Light	
36 Minutes PACED Cardio				

PHASE 8 – WORKOUT 3: SHOULDERS and ABS (Obliques)

WORKOUTS	SETS	REPS	WEIGHT REC-OMMENDED	WEIGHT USED
SM Behind Neck Press	4	8	80% 10RM	
DB Arnold Press	3	25	Light	
Trap Bar Shrug	3	25	Light	

Lateral Raises	4	25*	Light	
Front Raises	3	25	50-55% 10RM	
Russian Twist	4	25	Body	
Standing DB Oblique Crunch	4	25	Light	

PHASE 8 – WORKOUT 4: ARMS and 37 Minutes Cardio

WORKOUTS	SETS	REPS	WEIGHT REC-OMMENDED	WEIGHT USED
Close Grip Bench Press	4	15	Light-Medium	
Barbell Curl	4	25	Light	
Triceps Cable Pushdown	4	25	Light	
DB Kickbacks	3	25	Light	
Standing Dumb-bell Curls	3	25	Light	
Concentration Curl	3	25	Light	

37 Minutes PACED Cardio				

PHASE 8 – WORKOUT 5: LEGS and ABS (Mid/Top)

WORKOUTS	SETS	REPS	WEIGHT REC- OMMENDED	WEIGHT USED
Leg Press	2/5	6	85% 10RM	
Dumbbell Lunge	3	25	Light	
Goblet Squat	4	25	Light	
SM Calf Raises	4	25	Light	
Leg Curls	4	25*	Light-Medium	
Toe Touches	4	25		
Crunches	3	50		

PHASE 8 – WORKOUT 6: FULL BODY and 38 Minutes Cardio

WORKOUTS	SETS	REPS	WEIGHT REC-OMMENDED	WEIGHT USED
Barbell Row (underhand grip) ---superset--- Rear Delt Fly	2/4 4	6 25	85% 1RM Light	
Decline Bench Press	4	25	50-555% 1RM	
Leg Extensions	4	25	Light	
Upright Row (EZ-Bar)	4	25	Light	
38-Minute PACED Cardio				

HOW TO CREATE YOUR OWN PLAN

Due to the fact that I am unable to individually speak with everyone who purchases this book, I cannot accommodate for variables that exist in the development of the suggested programs. Every person and their circumstances are different. Whether you have an injury or you simply lack the equipment to complete said exercises, you can alter any plan to make up for the exercises you are unable to complete.

When constructing a workout plan, first, you want to do your compound movements. This is a multi-joint exercise which is usually the heaviest lift performed per workout session. These exercises require the most energy, so it is best to do them first. The second should be a static movement, which is a movement that involves your stabilizer muscles. This movement usually is performed on one side of the body at a time (such as a dumbbell press). Following the static lifts, you should perform your machine lifts.

These lifts have a specific range and path of motion every set. When your muscles are fatigued, the best way to ensure they are being activated properly is by using machines tailored to that body part. Lastly, are free weight exercises and cables. At the end of your workout, you can use these exercises to stress the muscle to full exhaustion and concentrate on its contractions. Due to the weight not being a factor, you should take the time to squeeze the muscle to get the best results.

The rep range should fall within whatever goal it is that you are trying to reach. 4-8 constitute as strength training, 8-12 is muscle hypotrophy and 12-20 is muscle endurance. Try to remember that as you increase the weight, you need to decrease the reps and vice versa. The number of sets should fall in line with the volume of the total workout.

PHASE 1 – WORKOUT 1: _____

WORKOUTS	SETS	REPS	WEIGHT REC-OMMENDED	WEIGHT USED

PHASE 1 – WORKOUT 2: _____

WORKOUTS	SETS	REPS	WEIGHT REC-OMMENDED	WEIGHT USED

PHASE 1 – WORKOUT 3: _____

WORKOUTS	SETS	REPS	WEIGHT REC-OMMENDED	WEIGHT USED

PHASE 1 – WORKOUT 4: _____

WORKOUTS	SETS	REPS	WEIGHT REC-OMMENDED	WEIGHT USED

PHASE 1 – WORKOUT 5: _____

WORKOUTS	SETS	REPS	WEIGHT REC-OMMENDED	WEIGHT USED

PHASE 1 – WORKOUT 6: _____

WORKOUTS	SETS	REPS	WEIGHT REC-OMMENDED	WEIGHT USED

PHASE 2 – WORKOUT 1: _____

WORKOUTS	SETS	REPS	WEIGHT REC-OMMENDED	WEIGHT USED

PHASE 2 – WORKOUT 2: _____

WORKOUTS	SETS	REPS	WEIGHT REC-OMMENDED	WEIGHT USED

PHASE 1 – WORKOUT 3:

WORKOUTS	SETS	REPS	WEIGHT REC-OMMENDED	WEIGHT USED

PHASE 2 – WORKOUT 4: _____

WORKOUTS	SETS	REPS	WEIGHT REC-OMMENDED	WEIGHT USED

PHASE 2 – WORKOUT 5: _____

WORKOUTS	SETS	REPS	WEIGHT REC-OMMENDED	WEIGHT USED

PHASE 2 – WORKOUT 6:

WORKOUTS	SETS	REPS	WEIGHT REC-OMMENDED	WEIGHT USED

PHASE 3 – WORKOUT 1: _____

WORKOUTS	SETS	REPS	WEIGHT REC-OMMENDED	WEIGHT USED

PHASE 3 – WORKOUT 2: _____

WORKOUTS	SETS	REPS	WEIGHT REC-OMMENDED	WEIGHT USED

PHASE 3 – WORKOUT 3: _____

WORKOUTS	SETS	REPS	WEIGHT REC-OMMENDED	WEIGHT USED

PHASE 3 – WORKOUT 4:

WORKOUTS	SETS	REPS	WEIGHT REC-OMMENDED	WEIGHT USED

PHASE 3 – WORKOUT 5:

WORKOUTS	SETS	REPS	WEIGHT REC-OMMENDED	WEIGHT USED

PHASE 3 – WORKOUT 6: _____

WORKOUTS	SETS	REPS	WEIGHT REC-OMMENDED	WEIGHT USED

PHASE 4 – WORKOUT 1: _____

WORKOUTS	SETS	REPS	WEIGHT REC-OMMENDED	WEIGHT USED

PHASE 4 – WORKOUT 2: _____

WORKOUTS	SETS	REPS	WEIGHT REC-OMMENDED	WEIGHT USED

PHASE 4 – WORKOUT 3: _____

WORKOUTS	SETS	REPS	WEIGHT REC-OMMENDED	WEIGHT USED

PHASE 4 – WORKOUT 4: _____

WORKOUTS	SETS	REPS	WEIGHT REC-OMMENDED	WEIGHT USED

PHASE 4 – WORKOUT 5: _____

WORKOUTS	SETS	REPS	WEIGHT REC-OMMENDED	WEIGHT USED

PHASE 4 – WORKOUT 6: _____

WORKOUTS	SETS	REPS	WEIGHT REC-OMMENDED	WEIGHT USED

PHASE 5 – WORKOUT 1:

WORKOUTS	SETS	REPS	WEIGHT RECOMMENDED	WEIGHT USED

PHASE 5 – WORKOUT 2:

WORKOUTS	SETS	REPS	WEIGHT RECOMMENDED	WEIGHT USED

PHASE 5 – WORKOUT 3:

WORKOUTS	SETS	REPS	WEIGHT REC-OMMENDED	WEIGHT USED

PHASE 5 – WORKOUT 4: _____

WORKOUTS	SETS	REPS	WEIGHT REC-OMMENDED	WEIGHT USED

PHASE 5 – WORKOUT 5: _____

WORKOUTS	SETS	REPS	WEIGHT REC-OMMENDED	WEIGHT USED

PHASE 5 – WORKOUT 6: _____

WORKOUTS	SETS	REPS	WEIGHT REC-OMMENDED	WEIGHT USED

PHASE 6 – WORKOUT 1: _____

WORKOUTS	SETS	REPS	WEIGHT REC-OMMENDED	WEIGHT USED

PHASE 6 – WORKOUT 2: _____

WORKOUTS	SETS	REPS	WEIGHT REC-OMMENDED	WEIGHT USED

PHASE 6 – WORKOUT 3: _____

WORKOUTS	SETS	REPS	WEIGHT REC-OMMENDED	WEIGHT USED

PHASE 6 – WORKOUT 4: _____

WORKOUTS	SETS	REPS	WEIGHT REC-OMMENDED	WEIGHT USED

PHASE 6 – WORKOUT 5: _____

WORKOUTS	SETS	REPS	WEIGHT REC-OMMENDED	WEIGHT USED

PHASE 6 – WORKOUT 6: _____

WORKOUTS	SETS	REPS	WEIGHT REC-OMMENDED	WEIGHT USED

PHASE 7 – WORKOUT 1: _____

WORKOUTS	SETS	REPS	WEIGHT REC-OMMENDED	WEIGHT USED

PHASE 7 – WORKOUT 2: _____

WORKOUTS	SETS	REPS	WEIGHT REC-OMMENDED	WEIGHT USED

PHASE 7 – WORKOUT 3:

WORKOUTS	SETS	REPS	WEIGHT REC- OMMENDED	WEIGHT USED

PHASE 7 – WORKOUT 4: _____

WORKOUTS	SETS	REPS	WEIGHT REC-OMMENDED	WEIGHT USED

PHASE 7 – WORKOUT 5: _____

WORKOUTS	SETS	REPS	WEIGHT REC-OMMENDED	WEIGHT USED

PHASE 7 – WORKOUT 6: _____

WORKOUTS	SETS	REPS	WEIGHT REC-OMMENDED	WEIGHT USED

PHASE 8 – WORKOUT 1: _____

WORKOUTS	SETS	REPS	WEIGHT REC-OMMENDED	WEIGHT USED

PHASE 8 – WORKOUT 2: _____

WORKOUTS	SETS	REPS	WEIGHT REC-OMMENDED	WEIGHT USED

PHASE 8 – WORKOUT 3: _____

WORKOUTS	SETS	REPS	WEIGHT REC-OMMENDED	WEIGHT USED

PHASE 8 – WORKOUT 4: _____

WORKOUTS	SETS	REPS	WEIGHT REC-OMMENDED	WEIGHT USED

PHASE 8 – WORKOUT 5: _____

WORKOUTS	SETS	REPS	WEIGHT REC-OMMENDED	WEIGHT USED

PHASE 8 – WORKOUT 6:

WORKOUTS	SETS	REPS	WEIGHT REC-OMMENDED	WEIGHT USED

END-OF-BOOK TIPS

—⚬◦◦—

10 Tips to Break Your Plateau

Switch your routine/split. Your body may be accustomed to your program.

Try different exercises. Instead of using a barbell, use machines and dumbbells.

Execute the lift using different grips. Go wider or closer than normal to activate different muscle fibers.

Use your spotter. Do not be afraid to do that extra rep.

Stick to a program long enough to see results.

Get more sleep.

After each set, flex and hold a contraction. Posing helps push blood to the area being worked.

Add more reps or weight. Increase the total volume of the workout.

Read. Be informed on your goal and how to reach it.

Go HARDER. Increase your focus in the gym. Use mind-muscle connection.

10 Tips to Build Muscle

Use a majority of compound movements to release more testosterone.

Time under tension. Slow down. Stop rushing through your set just to say you've completed the reps. The longer your muscle stress, the greater the response.

Add negative reps to your program. Descend the weight at a slower pace than normal.

Add pause reps to your program. At the bottom of the lift, pause for about 1-2 seconds.

Shorten your rest periods. If your break is too long, you may lose the pump.

Get out of your comfort zone. Stop doing only what it is you can do comfortably.

Add drop-sets to your program. This increases the total volume of the workout.

Strengthen your diet. Eat cleaner and increase your protein intake. A calorie surplus will lead to some good weight gains.

Change to a 3 and 1 split to target all muscle groups 2 times a week as opposed to 1.

Reduce your cardio. Though cardio is good, it can hinder progress when trying to add mass. Retain your calories.

10 Tips to Shred Body Fat

Decrease your calorie count.

Increase your cardio. Doing cardio more often will lead to burning more body fat.

Increase your repetitions. 12-15 is good but sometimes, going to 20 is great.

Don't fear the "small syndrome". Don't worry about what the scale says. If you look good, then that is the objective.

Decrease your carb intake post-workout. Your body will use fat as energy with no carbs available.

Drink more water. You should consume at least a gallon a day.

Do fewer compound movements and more static lifts. Also, you can implement H.I.I.T exercises to accelerate fat burning.

Find someone to hold you accountable. It will be even better if they want to shed a couple of pounds too.

Stop consuming calories after a certain time of the day. This may be seen as intermittent fasting.

Practice doing vacuums. Exhale all of the air in your lungs, and suck in your stomach, holding it for about 20 seconds. Do this about 4 times in a row every day.

www.ingramcontent.com/pod-product-compliance
Lightning Source LLC
Chambersburg PA
CBHW051717020426
42333CB00014B/1029